W9-CBA-871

Percutaneous Device Closure of the Atrial Septum

Percutaneous Device Closure of the Atrial Septum

Editor

Stephen J D Brecker MD FRCP FESC FACC
Consultant Cardiologist
Director, Cardiac Catheterisation Laboratories
St George's Hospital
London
UK

Foreword by

Bernard J Gersh MB ChB DPhil

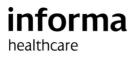

informa
healthcare

© 2006 Informa UK Limited

First published in the United Kingdom in 2006 by Informa Healthcare, 4 Park Square, Milton Park, Abingdon, Oxon OX14 4RN. Informa Healthcare is a trading division of Informa UK Ltd, Registered Office: 37/41 Mortimer Street, London, W1T 3JH. Registered in England and Wales Number 1072954.

Tel: +44 (0)20 7017 6000
Fax: +44 (0)20 7017 6699
Email: info.medicine@tandf.co.uk
Website: www.informahealthcare.com

All rights reserved. No part of this publication may be reproduced, stored in a retrieval system, or transmitted, in any form or by any means, electronic, mechanical, photocopying, recording, or otherwise, without the prior permission of the publisher or in accordance with the provisions of the Copyright, Designs and Patents Act 1988 or under the terms of any licence permitting limited copying issued by the Copyright Licensing Agency, 90 Tottenham Court Road, London W1P 0LP.

Although every effort has been made to ensure that all owners of copyright material have been acknowledged in this publication, we would be glad to acknowledge in subsequent reprints or editions any omissions brought to our attention.

Although every effort has been made to ensure that drug doses and other information are presented accurately in this publication, the ultimate responsibility rests with the prescribing physician. Neither the publishers nor the authors can be held responsible for errors or for any consequences arising from the use of information contained herein. For detailed prescribing information or instructions on the use of any product or procedure discussed herein, please consult the prescribing information or instructional material issued by the manufacturer.

A CIP record for this book is available from the British Library.

Library of Congress Cataloging-in-Publication Data
Data available on application

ISBN-10: 1 84184 596 5
ISBN-13: 978 1 84184 596 8

Distributed in North and South America by
Taylor & Francis
6000 Broken Sound Parkway, NW, (Suite 300)
Boca Raton, FL 33487, USA

Within Continental USA
Tel: 1 (800) 272 7737; Fax: 1 (800) 374 3401
Outside Continental USA
Tel: (561) 994 0555; Fax: (561) 361 6018
Email: orders@crcpress.com

Distributed in the rest of the world by
Thomson Publishing Services
Cheriton House
North Way
Andover, Hampshire SP10 5BE, UK
Tel: +44 (0)1264 332424
Email: tps.tandfsalesorder@thomson.com

Composition by J&L Composition, Filey, North Yorkshire
Printed and bound in Spain by Grafos SA Arte Sobre Papel

Dedication

To Lucy and Joshua

Contents

Contributors

Robert H Anderson BSc MD FRCPath
Joseph Levy Professor of Paediatric
Cardiac Morphology
Cardiac Unit
Institute of Child Health
University College London
London
UK

Franziska Büscheck
Medical student
CardioVascular Center Frankfurt
Sankt Katharinen
Frankfurt
Germany

Qi-Ling Cao MD
Congenital Heart Center
Depts Pediatrics and Medicine
University of Chicago Hospitals
Chicago, IL
USA

Paul Clift BSc MD MRCP
Consultant Cardiologist
Department of Cardiology
University Hospital
Birmingham NHS Foundation Trust
Birmingham
UK

Andrew C Cook MD
British Heart Foundation
Cardiac Unit
Institute of Child Health
London
UK

Anita Dumitrescu MD
Cardiology Consultant
Mater Misericordiae Hospital
Dublin
Ireland

Francisco Garay MD
Congenital Heart Center
Depts Pediatrics and Medicine
University of Chicago Hospitals
Chicago, IL
USA

Ziyad M Hijazi MD
George M Eisenberg Professor of
Pediatrics and Medicine
Congenital Heart Center
University of Chicago Hospitals
Chicago, IL
USA

Hugh S Markus FRCP
Professor of Neurology
Centre for Clinical Neuroscience
St George's University of London
London
UK

Michael J Mullen MD MRCP
Consultant Cardiologist
Royal Brompton Hospital
London
UK

Simon Nightingale FRCP
Consultant Neurologist
Royal Shrewsbury Hospital
Shrewsbury
UK

Igor F Palacios MD
Director of Interventional Cardiology
Massachusetts General Hospital
Harvard Medical School
Boston
USA

Rainer Schräder MD
Professor of
Medizische Klinik III-CCB
Markuskrankenhaus
Frankfurt am Main
Germany

Horst Sievert MD
Professor of Medicine
CardioVascular Center Frankfurt
Sankt Katharinen
Frankfurt
Germany

George R Sutherland BSc MB ChB FRCP
FESC
Professor of Cardiac Imaging
Dept of Cardiological Sciences
St George's Hospital Medical School
London
UK

Sara Thorne MD FRCP
Consultant Cardiologist
Department of Cardiology
University Hospital
Birmingham NHS Foundation Trust
Birmingham
UK

Kevin P Walsh MD
Cardiology Consultant
Mater Misericordae Hospital
Dublin
Ireland

Peter Wilmshurst FRCP
Consultant Cardiologist
Royal Shrewsbury Hospital
Shrewsbury
UK

Neil Wilson MD
Department of Paediatric Cardiology
John Radcliffe Hospital
Oxford
UK
and
Great Ormond Street Hospital
London
UK

Foreword

In patients without other structural heart disease, the persistence of a patent foramen ovale (PFO) into adulthood is well recognized as a common entity. The spectrum of interest has, however, shifted away from the concept of the PFO as an anatomical entity of minor clinical relevance to recognition that this may be responsible for several serious clinical conditions including paradoxical systemic embolism causing ischemic stroke and myocardial infarction, the platypnea-orthodeoxia syndrome, decompression sickness in divers, and complications following pulmonary embolism. The relationship between PFO and migraine and vascular headaches is not clearly understood but is the focus of a fascinating and ongoing story which could have implications for millions of patients around the world who have migraine headaches on a regular basis. Whether these patients are experiencing true migraine or just migraine-like symptoms (aura and headache) that are brought on by a secondary disease including PFO and paradoxical embolization is uncertain but will likely be clarified by ongoing trials.

The amenability of PFO to device closure has established a new frontier of percutaneous interventional cardiology and this has also been the stimulus for a variety of novel technologies which are now either in use or under development. Moreover, although the results of surgery for closure of an atrial septal defect are excellent, a percutaneous approach has provided an alternative approach which is now used in the majority of patients.

Given this background, this book is timely and highly topical. Dr Brecker has brought together an authoritative group of authors from both sides of the Atlantic and the resulting text is comprehensive and extremely up to date.

The first section of the book discusses the anatomy and clinical presentations of atrial septal defects in adults and the role of the PFO in cerebrovascular disease and diving-related decompression syndrome. Two very important chapters address in detail transthoracic and intracardiac imaging of the atrial septum.

The second section deals with the range of percutaneous closure methods currently available and provides a critical analysis of the advantages and limitations of a variety of devices, in addition to a general overview of closure technique. Ultimately, optimal technological innovations will rest upon a greater understanding of the pathology and pathophysiology of the patent foramen ovale and aortic stenosis at both a microscopic and cellular level. This will undoubtedly occur, but these advances will need to move in tandem with well-designed clinical trials. What are sorely needed are trials comparing device closure with medical therapy in regard to recurrent stroke in patients with prior cryptogenic stroke. Such trials are ongoing but the results will not be available for several years and, given the relatively low rates of recurrent stroke with either technique, the trials will require large numbers of patients in order to be adequately powered.

For the present, however, it is likely that increasing numbers of cardiologists from around the world will embark upon PFO closures, and there is a need for a comprehensive text covering the subject. This book fills that niche. Moreover, I would expect that the pace of change and the rapidly increasing body of knowledge in this area will ensure the need for further editions of this excellent book.

Bernard J Gersh MB ChB DPhil
Mayo Medical School
Rochester MN

Preface

The field of device closure of defects of the interatrial septum has expanded rapidly over the past ten years and it is likely that there will be further rapid increase in the numbers of procedures being performed. In this book we address the anatomy of the interatrial septum and review the types of defect that are amenable to device closure, including the patent foramen ovale. We review the imaging techniques that are available and the techniques used for closure. We have gathered together the world leaders in percutaneous closure to review the individual devices that are currently available. Each of the contributors has extensive experience in the use of these devices. We hope that this book will provide the interventional cardiologist with a useful resource with which to embark upon this important technique.

Acknowledgments

I would like to thank my colleague, Dr David Ward, with whom the device closure service was set up at St George's Hospital, London in 1998. His talents and inspiration have led to a successful partnership. I am of course indebted to the catheter lab nurses, cardiac physiologists and radiographers at St George's Hospital, London for their enthusiasm and assistance. I am grateful to Oliver Walter and Alan Burgess of Informa Healthcare for their assistance with this project, and the individual contributors, without whom it would not have been possible.

Section 1

Introduction

1

Anatomy of the atrial septum

Andrew C Cook

Introduction • The normal atrial septum • How should we describe the atrial septum?
• Interatrial communications within the oval fossa • Interatrial communications outside
the oval fossa • Conclusions

INTRODUCTION

For those wanting to perform device closure of the atrial septum, it is crucial to
have a good understanding of the anatomy of this region of the heart. Each
patient and each defect will have unique characteristics. Defects that allow interatrial shunting are sometimes found outside the confines of the atrial septum.
Being able to interpret morphology in unusual cases, therefore, requires not only
an understanding of normal anatomy but also an appreciation of the position of
defects relative to surrounding cardiac structures. Description of anatomy can
also become complicated if the heart is only considered in isolation and not in its
attitudinally correct position. As I will illustrate, most of such problems can now
be overcome by understanding the component parts that form the normal atrial
septum while also appreciating the position of those structures relative to the
body.

THE NORMAL ATRIAL SEPTUM

When one examines the structures separating the right from the left atrium in
anatomical specimens, there appears, at first, to be an extensive muscular wall
separating the two chambers (Figure 1.1). In fact, only a small proportion of this
musculature separates one atrium from the other. The remainder of the musculature is a series of folds between two adjacent structures. Appreciating the
different locations of these folds relative to the solid septal component is the key
to understanding the anatomy of the atrial septum.

Probably the best way to illustrate this is first to go back and look at the atrial
septum during fetal life. In the mid-gestation fetus, for instance, it is easy to
distinguish the middle part of the interatrial partition as a thin, mobile, pocket-
like structure when viewing the heart from its right or left atrial aspect (Figures
1.2a, b). This 'flap valve' is formed during embryonic development from the
primary atrial septum, which grows into and divides the initially common
atrium.[1] The upper margin of the primary septum subsequently breaks down to

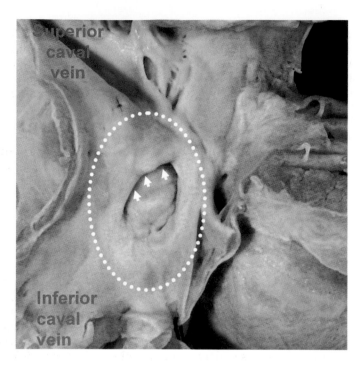

Figure 1.1　The normal atrial septum viewed from its right atrial aspect. On first inspection the septum appears as an extensive solid partition (dashed line) but in reality is a heterogeneous structure composed of a solid partition, surrounded by folds. Even when intact, there are often deep crevices within its superior, cranial margin (arrowheads).

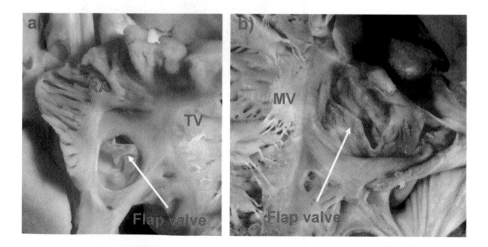

Figure 1.2　The atrial septum as seen in the mid-trimester fetus from the right atrium (a), and left atrium (b). At this stage of development, the mid portion can be distinguished easily as a thin pocket-like flap valve, which moves freely during the cardiac cycle during life. RA = right atrium; LA = left atrium; TV = tricuspid valve; MV = mitral valve.

form the 'ostium secundum', which forms the opening of the pocket. This inter-atrial communication, the opening of the pocket, is always placed initially in the cranial margin of the flap valve, in line with the direction of blood flow from the inferior caval vein. The rims, or limbus, of the oval foramen are formed slightly later during the first trimester of pregnancy, partly due to incorporation of the pulmonary veins into the left atrium and also by outward expansion of the atrial walls.[2] With time, the distinction between the flap valve and its rims becomes less obvious. Even during later gestation, the pocket-shaped flap valve becomes progressively straighter and less mobile with an increase in its muscular content.[3] As we know well, after birth it is then pushed against the left atrial side of its surrounding rims by the pressure of blood within the left atrium, fusing with them to varying degrees. There is variability in this maturation process between individuals, which in part may explain some of the variations in anatomy of the atrial septum found after birth and in adults. For example, in some newborns, and particularly in premature infants, the flap valve can retain its pocket-like configuration, even though it may be of sufficient size, completely to cover the rims of the oval foramen. In others, the amount of flap valvar tissue is excessive, such that it is aneurysmal and can then potentially obstruct the interatrial communication or inflows to the heart. These features can persist into adulthood but the oval fossa can also enlarge and become aneurysmal to a lesser degree, in the setting of atrial dilation. Although there is controversy about the significance of an aneurysmal atrial septum when seen in isolation, it is certainly encountered in some patients undergoing transcatheter closure of defects in the atrial septum (Figure 1.3).

The flap valve then, forms the oval fossa. It also forms the muscular rim of the oval fossa closest to the tricuspid valve but the structure of the oval fossa is quite

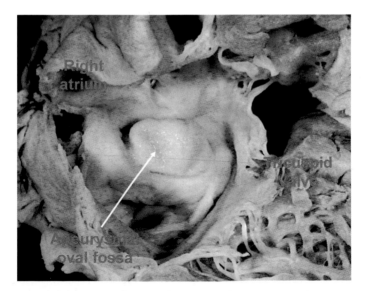

Figure 1.3 Example of an aneurysmal atrial septum. The part of the septum derived from the flap valve, the oval fossa, is dilated and bulges towards the right atrium in this specimen.

different from the majority of the 'rims' which surround it on its right side. The nature of these rims is perhaps best seen when looking at adult rather than fetal hearts, because by this time the folds have become filled with fatty tissue, which is easily distinguishable in anatomic specimens from muscle. Thus in cross section across the atrial septum, we can see that the rims are composed of two layers of atrial wall with fat in the middle (Figure 1.4). Although this dissection through the fossa will lead from one atrial cavity to the other (Figure 1.5a), and does not put the patient at immediate risk, perforation through the rims, will lead outside the heart into the fatty tissue which fills the folds and therefore into extracardiac space (Figure 1.5b). Thus dissection of the rims of the atrial septum is a dangerous situation potentially leading to cardiac tamponade. In addition, the fact that the structures that separate the right from left atrium are composed of the atrial septum, together with its surrounding rims, means that the partition cannot be considered a simple flat wall. Instead, it is important to remember that even in the normal situation, there are distinct rims projecting on its right atrial side. Often, and even in the setting of an intact atrial septum, there may be crevices or deep creases between the rims and the true atrial septum. Perforation

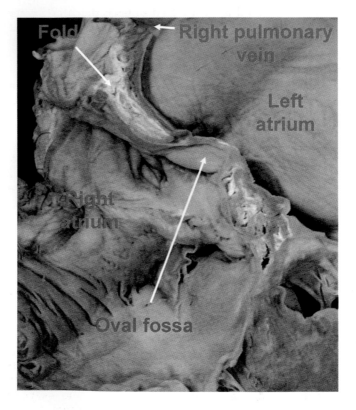

Figure 1.4   This section, across the atrial septum in an adult heart, shows the different components that make up the interatrial partition. The section is taken in a four-chamber plane. The oval fossa is seen as a solid partition, whereas the posterior rim comprises a fold of tissue between the right pulmonary veins and the right atrium, filled with fat.

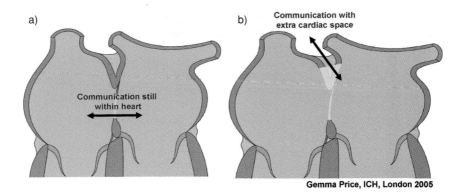

Figure 1.5   These schemes illustrate how perforation through the region of the oval fossa will lead from one atrium to the other (a). In contrast perforation through the posterior fold of tissue (b) will lead outside the heart and is potentially dangerous.

through these crevices could as easily lead outside the heart as into the left atrium.

HOW SHOULD WE DESCRIBE THE ATRIAL SEPTUM?

Having determined that the structure of the interatrial walls is heterogeneous, we then need some consistency in naming these structures. As will be discussed throughout this book, being able consistently to describe the location of defects within the atrial septum, as well as the nature of the rims surrounding the defects, is a crucial part of assessment prior to transcatheter closure. In our view, the nomenclature has become confused over time. In the past, it has been common for the anatomist, as least, to describe cardiac structures, including the atrial septum, as though the heart is sitting on its apex.[4] Thus, we have adopted many misnomers for cardiac structures which belie their true location within the body. As we know well, the right and left atriums and ventricles are in fact located anteriorly and posteriorly within the body, the left anterior descending coronary artery is superior, and the posterior descending coronary artery is inferior.[5] For the atrial septum, similar confusion exists. It is often not clear whether the superior rim, for example, refers to the upper rim with the heart sitting on its apex, or to the rim closest to the head with the heart in an attitudinally correct position. In order to circumvent these problems, we support the notion that it may be best to describe the atrial septum in terms of its relationship to surrounding cardiac structures while also then recognizing the location of these structures relative to the body co-ordinates.

Fortunately, the rims of the normal atrial septum hold a very close relationship to a number of easily recognizable cardiac landmarks. When viewing the rims from the right atrium, we can see, for example, that the most cranial rim is located immediately below the mouth of the superior caval vein and might, therefore, best be termed the superior caval rim. If one places an imaginary clockface on the right side of the atrium septum, this rim would extend from approximately 10 to 12 o'clock (Figure 1.6). In cross-section, it is seen to be a fold

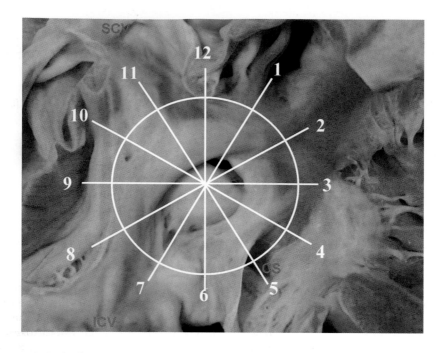

Figure 1.6   In this heart, viewed from the right atrial aspect, we have overlaid a clockface as an aid to describing the rims of the oval foramen.
SCV, superior caval vein; ICV, inferior caval vein; CS, coronary sinus; TV, tricuspid valve.

of myocardium between the superior caval vein and the left atrium. Opposite this rim, at 6 to 8 o'clock, we have the rim adjacent to the mouth of the inferior caval vein. This rim is often very small, so there will be continuity between the leftward wall of the inferior caval vein and the atrial septum. This can make it particularly difficult to distinguish defects within the inferior portion of the oval fossa from interatrial communications known as inferior sinus venosus defects. Nonetheless, this rim could justifiably be termed the inferior caval rim. There is then the fold which forms a rim at 12 to 2 o'clock situated behind the aortic root, a 'retro-aortic rim', and the rim situated adjacent to the pulmonary veins, the pulmonary venous rim. This latter rim, occupying the region from 7 to 10 o'clock, is a fold between the pulmonary veins and the right atrium or superior caval vein. It is also known as the secondary septum; externally it is marked by a deep crevice known as Sondergaard's or Waterston's groove. The final rims, situated adjacent to the triangle of Koch infero-anteriorly within the right atrium, are perhaps the most complicated. Inferiorly, at 4 to 6 o'clock, in the region of the mouth of the coronary sinus, the rim is formed of a fold between the inferior caval vein and coronary sinus, the so-called 'sinus septum', which carries on its crest the Eustachian valve or ridge. More cranially and medially, at about 2 to 4 o'clock on our imaginary clockface, and towards the apex of the triangle of Koch, the fold turns into a solid muscular structure which carries within it the tendon of Todaro, itself anchored to the central fibrous body. Thus the anterior rim of the atrial septum is a solid muscular structure separated from the triangle of Koch and atrioventricular septal structures by the tendon of Todaro. This latter rim is well recognized by the echocardiographer as the point of insertion of the aortic leaflet of the mitral valve when viewing the heart in four-chamber section.

INTERATRIAL COMMUNICATIONS WITHIN THE OVAL FOSSA

The patent oval foramen

From the preceding discussion, it is relatively easy to understand the situation in which the flap valve of the oval foramen overlaps the folds which surround it, but has failed to fuse completely with them, leading to a patent oval foramen. Usually in this situation, the potential communication between right and left atrium is found below the cranial rim of the atrial septum and corresponds to the opening in the flap valve during fetal life (Figure 1.7). More rarely it can be situated more towards the atrioventricular valvar, or pulmonary venous rims. The communication can take a tortuous course such that the opening on the right side of the atrial septum is not aligned with that on the left side. More frequently, the communication may have considerable length such that it forms a tunnel. This results when there is marked overlap between the flap valve and the rims of the atrial septum. Indeed, in this situation it can appear as though the left atrial opening of the tunnel reaches the roof of the left atrium. Both tortuous and tunnel variations of a patent oval foramen can impact on closure by

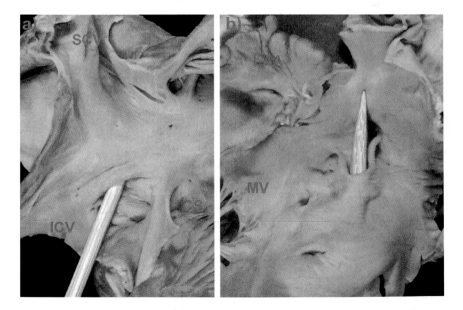

Figure 1.7 An example of a probe patent oval foramen in an adult viewed from the right (a) and left (b) atrial aspects. The flap valve in this specimen overlaps the rims of the oval foramen sufficiently but has failed to fuse with its cranial margin completely. This leads to a potential communication between the right and left atrium. SCV = superior caval vein; ICV = inferior caval vein; CS = coronary sinus; LAA = left atrial appendage; MV = mitral valve.

interventional means since they can potentially lead to abnormal orientation or anchoring of the device. Clearly, this will also depend on the design of the device bring used and the method of deployment.

Oval fossa defects

True atrial septal defects are then characterized by further deficiencies within the confines of the oval fossa. In the past, such defects have also been known as 'secundum defects' since they are present at the site of the secondary embryonic foramen, although it is worth noting from the preceding discussion that they are due to deficiencies in the primary atrial septum, not the secondary septum. This is our reasoning for choosing to call them oval fossa defects. Often, the deficiency is as a result of the flap valve, or its rims, being of insufficient size to overlap one another in the superior caval, or retroaortic margin (Figure 1.8). The 'rims', of the defect, seen echocardiographically, will then be the infolded wall of the oval fossa cranially and the solid partition forming the oval fossa inferiorly. Alternatively, there may be perforations within the body of the oval fossa, either solitary or multiple (Figure 1.9). In this situation, the apparent margins of the defect visible by ultrasound will consist of tissue derived from the oval fossa

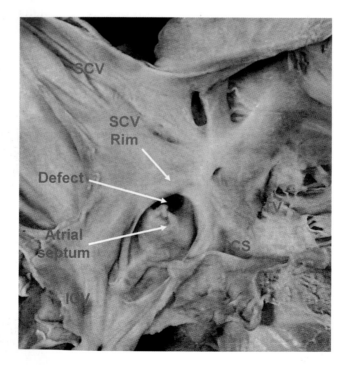

Figure 1.8 This oval fossa defect is solitary and situated within the cranial or superior caval margin, and is a result of the flap valve being too short to cover this rim completely. The superior rim of the defect is therefore formed from the fold between the superior caval vein and left atrium, while the inferior rim is formed from the tissue of the atrial septum. SCV = superior caval vein; ICV = inferior caval vein; CS = coronary sinus; TV = tricuspid valve.

and not to the infolded rims of the oval fossa itself. Depending on the muscularization of this tissue during development, the support provided for device placement will vary. Of particular note, such holes within the oval fossa are commonly oval, rather than circular, making assessment by echocardiography, using multiple planes of interrogation important, or else balloon sizing necessary. At the extreme end of the spectrum most of the atrial septum can be missing, or else perforated with only a mesh of septal remnants remaining (Figures 1.10, 1.11). In this situation, the margins of the defect seen echocardiographically will then approximate to the true rims of the oval fossa. When the oval fossa defects are large, there may be additional effacement of the surrounding rims. Although the conduction tissue would be in its anticipated normal position, originating from the apex of the triangle of Koch, in the situation of marked effacement of the anterior rim, only a narrow strip of muscle remains between the defect and the apex of the triangle of Koch and therefore the atrioventricular node may be more at risk from placement of devices (Figure 1.12). In contrast, in the setting of a dilated coronary sinus, the triangle of Koch will be broader than usual, and the tendon of Todaro rotated around the central fibrous body, from its near vertical position into a more horizontal plane. This effectively displaces the atrial septum cranially (Figure 1.13).

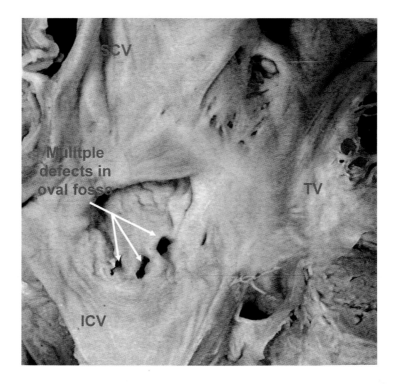

Figure 1.9   In this heart, again viewed from the right atrium, there are three small defects within the inferior, or caudal margin of the oval fossa, close to the mouth of the inferior caval vein. SCV = superior caval vein; ICV = inferior caval vein; CS = coronary sinus; TV = tricuspid valve.

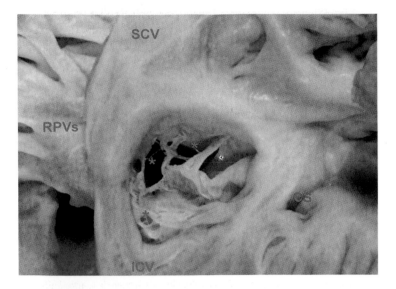

Figure 1.10   In this heart, the flap valve is not muscularized and has retained its membranous form, similar to that seen in fetal life. There are multiple perforations within the body of the flap valve, leaving a web of tissue separating the right and left atriums. SCV = superior caval vein; ICV = inferior caval vein; CS = coronary sinus; TV = tricuspid valve; RPVs = right pulmonary veins.

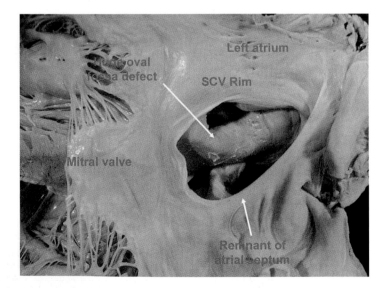

Figure 1.11   A huge defect within the oval fossa is shown from the left side of an adult specimen. There is virtually no true atrial septum present, and as a result, the margins of the defect approximate the rims of the oval fossa. SCV = superior caval vein.

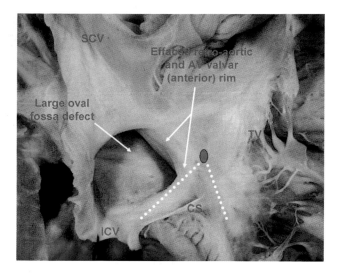

Figure 1.12   An example of a large oval fossa defect in which there is marked effacement of the rims closest to the atrioventricular valves and aortic root. As a result, there is a relatively narrow strip of musculature remaining between the defect and the atrioventricular node (green oval) which is situated at the cranial apex of the triangle of Koch (dashed lines). SCV = superior caval vein; ICV = inferior caval vein; CS = coronary sinus; TV = tricuspid valve.

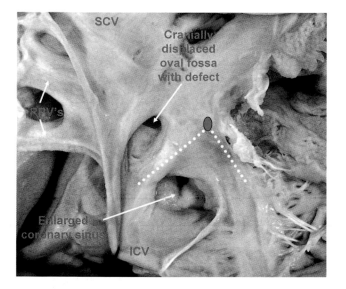

Figure 1.13   In this heart, viewed from the right atrium, there is enlargement of the coronary sinus in association with a persistent left superior caval vein. Since the coronary sinus forms the base of Koch's triangle, the triangle (dashed lines) is also broader than usual. As a result, the oval fossa, containing a small defect, is displaced cranially. Note the greater distance in this specimen between the defect and the atrioventricular node (green oval). SCV = superior caval vein; ICV = inferior caval vein; CS = coronary sinus; TV = tricuspid valve; RPVs = right pulmonary veins.

INTERATRIAL COMMUNICATIONS OUTSIDE THE OVAL FOSSA

From the preceding discussion, it will be apparent that the majority of interatrial communications are found within the confines of the oval fossa. Defects can exist, nonetheless, such that there is potential for interatrial shunting outside these margins. It is as important for the interventionist, as it is for the surgeon, to recognize these defects since there are commonly associated anomalies of the pulmonary veins, coronary sinus or atrioventricular valves that usually make them far less amenable to closure by transcatheter means.

Interatrial communications related to the mouths of the superior or inferior caval veins – 'sinus venosus defects'

The first of these defects, 'sinus venosus' interatrial communications, is best considered as an abnormal communication between the atriums, behind Sondergaard's or Waterston's groove (Figure 1.14). As described already, this fold of tissue, the secondary septum, normally separates the right pulmonary veins from the right atrium and forms relatively late in embryonic development only after incorporation of the pulmonary veins into the left atrium.[2] A channel through this groove, effectively results in anomalous connection of the right pulmonary veins to both the right and the left atrium, as well as an interatrial communication (Figures 1.15, 1.16). Although rare, such defects are more often located close to the mouth of the superior rather than inferior caval vein. The mouth of the superior caval vein will then override the remaining superior

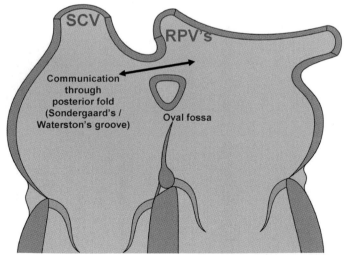

Gemma Price, ICH, London 2005

Figure 1.14   This diagram shows the essence of a sinus venosus defect. The defect represents an abnormal channel within the fold of tissue that normally separates the right pulmonary veins from the right atrium (Sondergaard's or Waterston's groove). The resulting interatrial communication is therefore outside the confines of the oval fossa and the right pulmonary veins are connected to both right and left atriums. SCV = superior caval vein; RPVs = right pulmonary veins.

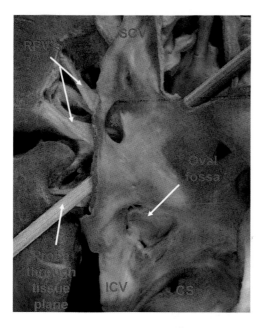

Figure 1.15 An example of a superior sinus venosus defect is shown from the right atrial aspect. The defect (∗) is separated from the oval fossa by a tissue plane through which a probe has been placed. The mouth of the superior caval vein overrides the cranial margin of the defect and the right upper pulmonary veins override its posterior aspect. SCV = superior caval vein; ICV = inferior caval vein; CS = coronary sinus; RPVs = right pulmonary veins.

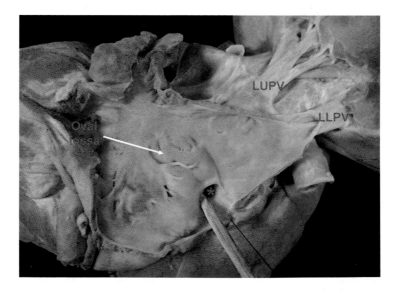

Figure 1.16 View of the same specimen as in Figure 1.15 from the left atrium. Again the sinus venosus defect (∗) can be seen as an interatrial communication outside the confines of the oval fossa, and is also unrelated to the left pulmonary veins. LAA = left atrial appendage; LUPV = left upper pulmonary vein; LLPV = left lower pulmonary vein.

rim of the oval fossa to varying degrees. Indeed, a tissue plane can be found between the oval fossa itself and the defect (Figure 1.15). In the setting of an inferior defect, the posteroinferior rim of the oval fossa will override the inferior caval vein to varying degrees. Since this rim is usually small, it can be hard to distinguish these types of interatrial communication from inferiorly located oval fossa defects, solely by their position (Figure 1.9). In our view, the key to differentiating the two is the anomalous connection of the lower right pulmonary veins, which is only found in the setting of a defect of the inferior sinus venosus type. More recently, we have seen two examples in which there was minimal overriding of the caval veins, but undoubtedly the defect is of the sinus venosus type and outside the region of the true atrial septum. This confirms to us that it is anomalous sharing of the pulmonary veins between the two atriums which is the key feature in this malformation. Closure of these defects via device placement would be difficult. Since there is usually overriding of a caval vein, the device would need to be shaped, or placed obliquely across the defect without obstructing either the path to the systemic, or the right pulmonary veins. As the posterior wall of the defect is effectively formed by the right pulmonary veins (Figure 1.15), there is also little in the way of rim to the defect in this region.

Interatrial communications via the mouth of the coronary sinus

Abnormal communications between the walls of the coronary sinus and the left atrium can also lead to an interatrial communication, but via the mouth of the coronary sinus. In this situation, it is important to note that the defect is inferior within the right atrium and once again outside the region of the true atrial septum. Often referred to as 'unroofing' of the coronary sinus, this is, once again, not anatomically correct. It has now been established that the coronary sinus has its own discrete walls from the outset of development, although fibers from the left atrial myocardium can insert into and envelop these walls.[6] Thus, unroofing of the coronary sinus would lead not into the left atrium but into extracardiac space. Instead, the communication is perhaps better likened to an abnormal conduit between the coronary sinus and left atrium. This can be of varying dimensions. The spectrum ranges from one or more small fenestrations (Figure 1.17), to a communication extending the entire length of the coronary sinus (Figures 1.18, 1.19). There is then usually marked dilation of the mouth of the coronary sinus and persistence of a left superior caval vein, which will enter the roof of the left atrium between the left atrial appendage and the left pulmonary veins. Once again, this is a difficult lesion to close by interventional means. Although small fenestrations potentially could be closed, larger communications would likely require closure of the mouth of the coronary sinus. When dilated, the mouth of the coronary sinus frequently occupies a large proportion of the triangle of Koch. It encroaches, anterosuperiorly, on the region of the atrioventricular node, anteriorly, onto the tricuspid valve, and

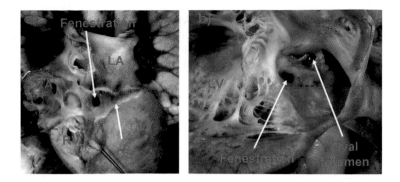

Figure 1.17 This fetal specimen shows a fenestration between the coronary sinus and the left atrium. When viewed from beneath (a) with the coronary sinus opened along its length, a small hole can be seen within the course of the coronary sinus. From the left atrial aspect (b) the opening into the left atrium can be seen and is outside the region of the oval fossa. RA = right atrium; RV = right ventricle; LA = left atrium; LV = left ventricle; CS = coronary sinus.

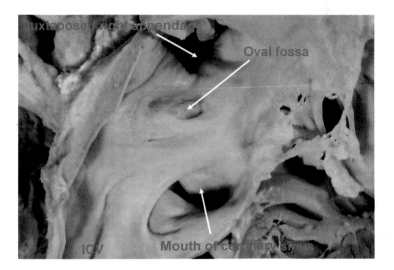

Figure 1.18 An example of an interatrial communication through the mouth of the coronary sinus, viewed from the right atrial aspect. In this heart the coronary sinus is enlarged and the oval fossa is intact. There is also juxtaposition of the right appendage. ICV = inferior caval vein.

posteroinferiorly, onto the fold separating it from the inferior caval vein. All of these structures could therefore be affected by device placement. Anomalous connection of a left superior caval vein to the roof of the left atrium would also need to be addressed.

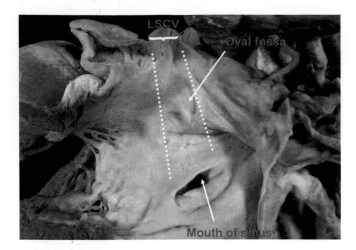

Figure 1.19   The left atrial aspect of the same heart as shown in Figure 1.18 shows that the communication is large and inferior to the oval fossa. In contrast to the example shown in Figure 1.17, most of the walls of the coronary sinus are absent (dashed lines). LSCV = left superior caval vein.

Ostium primum atrial septal defects

The final types of defect that need to be distinguished from deficiencies of the oval fossa are the so-called ostium primum atrial septal defects. Once again this is a misnomer since the essence of this malformation is not deficiency of the atrial septum but of the atrioventricular septal structures. This malformation is, therefore, one of the forms of atrioventricular septal defect with a common atrioventricular junction. The structure of the atrioventricular valves will reflect this, and not be those of a normal tricuspid or mitral valve.[7] In this condition, there is, of course, persistence of the embryonic ostium primum, since it is closure of this aperture by coalescence of the atrioventricular cushions, vestibular spine, ventricular and atrial septums, that sets the scene for formation of the atrioventricular septal sandwich.[8] The potential for shunting of blood is also often considered to be 'at atrial level' as it occurs above the level of the atrioventricular valves, which in this malformation are fused together in their mid-portion and to the crest of the ventricular septum (Figure 1.20). In most instances, nonetheless, closer inspection shows that the communication between the two atriums is below the level of the atrioventricular junction through the region normally occupied by the atrioventricular septum.[9] Closure of this form of interatrial communication by a device is likely to be fraught with difficulties, not only because of the abnormal structure of the atrioventricular valves, but also in view of the close proximity of the hole to the atrioventricular valves and ventricular conduction tissues.

CONCLUSIONS

We have shown how the structure of the normal atrial septum is heterogeneous and its margins are closely related to many other cardiac components. Defects

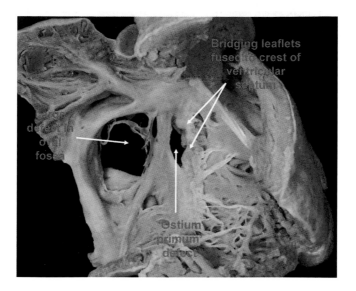

Figure 1.20 This specimen shows the essence of the so-called ostium primum atrial septal defect. In reality, this defect is one form of an atrioventricular septal defect with common atrioventricular junction, and is therefore outside the region of the true atrial septum, or oval fossa. Since the bridging leaflets are fused to each other, and to the crest of the ventricular septum, shunting of blood is above the level of valvar leaflets and often considered to be at atrial level. Closer inspection shows that the defect itself, and therefore level of shunting, crosses the plane of the atrioventricular junction. In this heart, there is also a huge fenestrated oval fossa defect. RA = right atrium; RV = right ventricle.

are usually confined to the oval fossa but the nature of the margins, or rims, will vary depending on the location, size, and number of holes. Interatrial communications can also exist outside the region of the oval fossa. The anatomy in these situations is far more complex and far less amenable to transcatheter closure.

REFERENCES

1. Anderson RH, Brown NA, Webb S. Development and structure of the atrial septum. Heart 2002; 88(1):104–10.
2. Webb S, Kanani M, Anderson RH, Richardson MK, Brown NA. Development of the human pulmonary vein and its incorporation in the morphologically left atrium. Cardiol Young 2001; 11(6):632–42.
3. Firpo C, Zielinsky P. Mobility of the flap valve of the primary atrial septum in the developing human fetus. Cardiol Young 1998; 8(1):67–70.
4. Beerman LB, Zuberbuhler JR. Atrial septal defect. In Paeditatric Cardiology 2nd Ed. Anderson RH, Baker EJ, Macartney FJ, Rigby ML, Shinebourne E, Tynan M (eds). London, Churchill Livingstone, 2002; 901–30.
5. Cook AC, Anderson RH. Attitudinally correct nomenclature. Heart 2002; 87(6):503–6.
6. Knauth A, McCarthy KP, Webb S et al. Interatrial communication through the mouth of the coronary sinus. Cardiol Young 2002; 12(4):364–72.

7. Anderson RH, Ho SY, Falcao S, Deliento L, Rigby ML. The diagnostic features of atrioventricular septal defect with common atrioventricular junction. Cardiol Young 1998; 8: 33–49.
8. Anderson RH, Webb S, Brown NA, Lamers W, Moorman A. Development of the heart: (2) Septation of the atriums and ventricles. Heart 2003; 89(8):949–58.
9. Falcao S, Daliento L, Ho SY, Rigby ML, Anderson RH. Cross sectional echocardiographic assessment of the extent of the atrial septum relative to the atrioventricular junction in atrioventricular septal defect. Heart 1999; 81(2):199–205.

2

Clinical presentation of the atrial septal defect in adults

Paul Clift and Sara Thorne

Introduction • Embryology of the interatrial septum • Presenting symptoms
• Examination findings • Investigations • Conclusions

INTRODUCTION

The early cardiologists were much perplexed with the diagnosis and clinical presentation of an atrial septal defect. The appearance of the patient was given a prominence not seen today. A typical patient would have 'a gracile habitus, arachnodactyly, high arched palate, and praecordial bulge',[1] whereas modern cardiologists would associate the above as signs of Marfan's disease. The predominant presenting feature then as now is breathlessness on exertion but this occurs later in adult life commonly in the third decade and is inconsistent and nonspecific. Many patients are asymptomatic and their defects are picked up on routine examination, either because of clinical demonstration of a murmur with associated features of right heart volume load, or from chest radiograph (CXR) appearances. This text will discuss briefly the relevant anatomy and embryology, also the ways in which atrial septal defects (ASD) present, and the physical signs and relevant clinical investigations used in making the diagnosis.

EMBRYOLOGY OF THE INTERATRIAL SEPTUM

In order to understand why there are a variety of atrial septal defects it is worth reviewing the embryological development of the inter atrial septum.

In the first eight weeks of embryological life the heart is formed. Initially the heart tube develops into a primitive ventricle with a common atrium above it. In the roof of this atrium the truncus arteriosus causes an indentation which will eventually become the secundum septum.

How an atrioventricular septal defect occurs

Partitioning of the atrium into left and right atria begins with the formation of the septum primum. This septum moves forward towards the endocardial cushions which will eventually form the orifices of the atrioventricular valves; the leading edge of the septum primum marks the margin of the ostium primum. Failure of the endocardial cushions to form leads to persistence of the ostium primum part of the complex anomaly, the atrioventricular septal defect.

How a secundum atrial septal defect occurs

Before fusion of the septum primum and endocardial cushions occurs, perforations appear in the septum primum allowing continuation of flow across the atrial septum; these coalesce to form the ostium secundum. The secundum septum is a passive down folding of the groove formed by the truncus arteriosus in the roof of the atria. It moves downwards and its leading edge forms the margins of the fossa ovalis. This persists to allow the normal flow of blood through the right atrium and into the left atrium in fetal life. Following birth and the act of breathing, the pulmonary venous return increases the pressure in the left atrium pushing the septum primum across onto the secundum septum closing the fossa ovalis. The septums then fuse together. Failure of this to occur results in a patent foramen ovale. Failure of the septum primum or secundum to overlap leads to a secundum defect. Ostium primum defects only occur in the context of an atrioventricular septal defect.

The patent foramen ovale (PFO) is found in around one fifth of the population and is a normal variant. It may present in the context of paradoxical embolic phenomena, such as stroke, transient ischemic attacks, or distal emboli. It is also implicated in the decompression illness that may affect divers following ascent from dives, as is discussed in later chapters.

How a sinus venosus defect occurs

The left and right sinus horns of the sinus venosus differentiate into the coronary sinus that runs along the floor of the left atrium, and the superior and inferior vena cavae that form the lateral wall of the right atrium. Defects can occur at the site of insertion of the sinus venosus into the right atrial cavity, with those in the superior aspect being associated with anomalous drainage of the right-sided pulmonary veins, so-called sinus venosus defects.[2] The coronary sinus defect occurs when the coronary sinus is unroofed allowing the pulmonary venous return to flow back to the right atrium. The sites of the various defects are represented in Figure 2.1.

PRESENTING SYMPTOMS

The presenting symptoms of any atrial communication depend on the size of the shunt (that is, the amount of blood passing from the left atrium into the right atrium). Small defects usually do not cause symptoms; however, moderate or large defects are associated with significant cardiovascular symptoms. The exertional dyspnea due to the left to right shunt is often misdiagnosed as asthma of childhood.

In an early reported series, an ASD was not considered to be benign; the reported mortality was 50% at 36 years and 10% at 60 years.[3] This early series dealt with patients diagnosed on chest radiograph and on clinical examination, so only the bigger defects were diagnosed; this clearly skews the survival data.

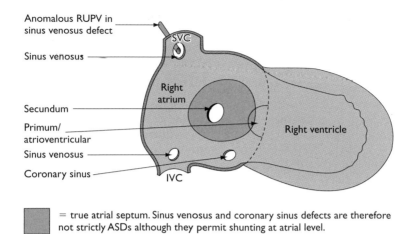

Anomalous RUPV in sinus venosus defect

SVC

Sinus venosus

Right atrium

Secundum

Primum/ atrioventricular

Sinus venosus

Coronary sinus

IVC

Right ventricle

= true atrial septum. Sinus venosus and coronary sinus defects are therefore not strictly ASDs although they permit shunting at atrial level.

Figure 2.1   Schematic representation of the various atrial septal defects.

The reported incidence of atrial septal defects has increased owing to improved diagnostic imaging. With current 2-dimensional and 3-dimensional transthoracic echocardiography with harmonics and contrast imaging, plus transesophageal echocardiography, the ability of the physician to correctly diagnose even the smallest ASD or PFO is far greater than that of the pioneering cardiologists of the mid 20th century.

Asymptomatic individual, an incidental finding

A truly incidental finding of an ASD is rare, but is usually made following the finding of a flow murmur through the pulmonary valve (often during pregnancy) and subsequent confirmation by transthoracic echocardiography. Although routine chest radiography is rarely carried out in the modern era, this may pick up an occasional atrial septal defect with classical radiographic signs, as described below.

Effort intolerance

In an original series of 62 adults with an ASD diagnosed on chest radiograph, with an average QP:QS of 2.5:1, the commonest presenting feature ($\sim$ 68%) was dyspnea on exertion or effort intolerance, with 21% being asymptomatic and 11% in heart failure.[1]

The left to right shunting will reduce the effective cardiac output and increase pulmonary blood flow on exertion leading to inadequate oxygen supply to the tissues; fatigue and dyspnea ensue. Indeed, adult patients with a hemodynamically significant ASD and normal pulmonary artery pressures have reduced cardiopulmonary performance.[4] Effort intolerance improves following closure of the defect both in terms of cardiopulmonary performance.[4-6] However, if there is significant pulmonary arterial hypertension (peak systolic PA pressure >50 mmHg) this improvement is not seen, indicating the importance of pulmonary arterial hypertension on long-term outcomes.[7] Older groups of patients also benefit in terms of symptomatic improvement in NYHA score.[8] Similar improvements in cardiopulmonary performance and NYHA score are seen following device closure of ASD in minimally symptomatic or asymptomatic adult patients of all ages,[6] associated with reduction in right ventricular dimensions.[9]

There is often mild elevation of the pulmonary artery pressure. However, severe pulmonary hypertension is rare and one should avoid classifying patients who are cyanotic with an ASD as having Eisenmenger's syndrome; the pulmonary arterial hypertension is more likely to be idiopathic. In patients over 50 years, even modest pulmonary hypertension (mean PA pressure >30 mmHg), is associated with less symptomatic improvement and greater risk of arrhythmias post surgical ASD closure.[10]

The decrease in left ventricular compliance that occurs with advancing age will further increase the left to right shunt, and combined with modest elevations of pulmonary artery pressure, will exacerbate the effort intolerance seen with an ASD. Rarely, a patient may present with heart failure as a consequence of the volume load and a failing right ventricle.

Neurological events

Whilst atrial septal defects are diagnosed in young adults with cryptogenic stroke disease, persistence of the foramen ovale is seen far more commonly. Up to 50% of young adults with a cryptogenic stroke, 21% with risk factors for stroke disease, and 40% with a single risk factor for stroke disease, have a PFO on bubble contrast echocardiography.[11] The causal relationship between PFO and stroke disease is poorly understood, however, there are two principal theories:

- An embolus arises from the systemic venous system and passes through the PFO when the right atrial pressure is transiently raised above the left atrial pressure such as occurs following a valsalva maneuver, during coughing or vigorous sniffing.
- The anatomy of the PFO may play a contributory role. The original flap valve of the foramen ovale may seal incompletely and leave a long tunnel-like flap between the right and left atria. Within this tunnel a clot may form, and this may be dislodged into the systemic circulation at times of higher right atrial pressure as described above.

In a recent meta-analysis of all the trial data on stroke prevention in patients with cryptogenic stroke and PFO, the event rate for recurrent strokes or transient ischemic attacks per 100 patient years is 4.2 (95% CI 3.4–5.0) for medical therapy ($n = 943$), 4.1 (95% CI 2.1–7.1) for surgical PFO closure ($n = 161$) and 1.6 (95% CI 1.1–2.2) for percutaneous device closure ($n = 1430$),[12] supporting a strategy of percutaneous device closure of PFOs in patients with cryptogenic stroke.

There are no data to support a strategy of routine PFO closure in the asymptomatic individual as a PFO is a normal variant in 10–20% of the general population. Similarly small (<0.5 cm in diameter) asymptomatic ASDs are unlikely to cause problems, and closure is not warranted.

Particular types of decompression illness in divers are associated with the presence of a potential right to left shunt at cardiac level, usually a patent foramen ovale; this is discussed in detail in a later chapter.

Arrhythmias

Palpitations are a common presenting feature of atrial septal defects. In patients with an ASD with right atrial dilatation, atrial arrhythmias will increase over time. This may be related to atrial electrical remodeling. This has been demonstrated in patients with a hemodynamically significant ASD with no history of arrhythmias.[13] These changes persist after closure of the defects and this may explain why patients[14] are still at risk of arrhythmias following device closure of their ASD.[15]

The age at which the defect is closed is important in predicting risk of future arrhythmias, with very few long-term sequelae if the ASD is closed in childhood.[16] The older the age at surgical repair the greater the risk of late arrhythmias,[17] with those over the age of 40 at greater risk than those below.[18]

Patients with arrhythmias and a suspected ASD should be put forward for defect closure; they should be anticoagulated with coumarins and rate controlled. Cardioversion is unlikely to be successful in the long term without closure of the defect, but should be attempted once the defect has been closed.

EXAMINATION FINDINGS

In a small ASD the cardiac examination may be entirely normal. The volume load on the right ventricle that occurs in larger defects leads to the typical examination findings. These are a right ventricular parasternal heave, a flow murmur through the pulmonary valve (not flow through the defect) and fixed splitting of the second heart sound. The widely split second sound is thought to occur due to delayed closure of the pulmonary valve due to the increased volume in the right heart. Fixed splitting of the second sound also occurs in patients with right bundle branch block or pulmonary stenosis. The patient may be in atrial fibrillation. Respiratory examination is unremarkable.

INVESTIGATIONS

ECG

There is often mild right axis deviation and mild prolongation of the QRS complex with a right bundle branch block pattern (Figure 2.2). The right bundle appears to function normally during electrophysiology studies in children despite the right bundle branch block pattern, which is thought to occur as a result of right ventricular volume loading.[19]

Atrial fibrillation occurs with increased frequency from the fourth decade onwards and is common by 60 years in unoperated patients. Atrial flutter can occur late after surgical repair and is often a scar-related macro re-entrant tachycardia (see Figure 2.2). Electrophysiology studies in patients with an ASD

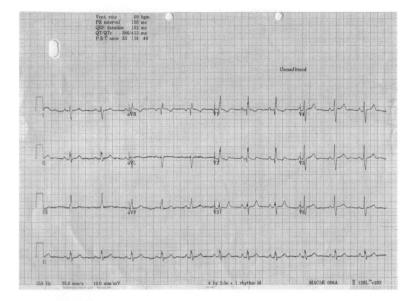

Figure 2.2 12-lead electrocardiogram of an adult male with a large secundum ASD and modest elevation of pulmonary artery pressures. There is incomplete right bundle branch block, right axis deviation, and evidence of right ventricular hypertrophy.

suggest that the right heart volume load leads to changes in sinus node and atrioventricular node function which normalize following closure of the defect. These changes occur as early as the third year of life.[20,21]

Chest radiography

Small atrial septal defects and patent foramen ovale may have a normal cardiac silhouette and pulmonary vascular markings. Larger defects with a significant left to right shunt classically have cardiomegaly with an increased cardiothoracic ratio (>50%). There is dilatation of the central pulmonary arteries and pulmonary plethora, the aortic knuckle may be small (Figure 2.3).

Echocardiography

In the adult, transthoracic echocardiography (TTE) may be diagnostic demonstrating a clearly visible defect in the atrial septum, best seen in the apical four-chamber and sub-costal long-axis views. However it is common to see 'echo fallout' in the region of the interatrial septum and this may lead to misdiagnosis of an ASD or incorrectly describing the ASD as 'echo fallout'. Improvements in two-dimensional (2D) echocardiography with harmonic imaging have improved the diagnostic accuracy of echocardiography.

A detailed discussion of the use of transthoracic and transesophageal echocardiography is given in a later chapter, but it is worth highlighting some key points regarding the use of these imaging modalities:

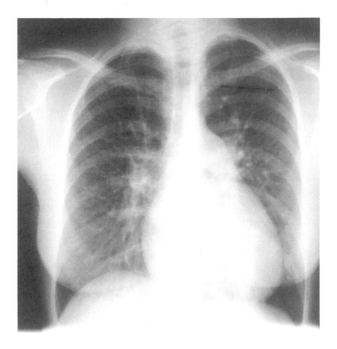

Figure 2.3   Chest radiograph of adult patient with large secundum atrial septal defect. Note the dilated heart, prominent central pulmonary arteries, pulmonary artery, and small aortic knuckle.

- Bubble contrast echocardiography with provocation has led to the accurate diagnosis of interatrial communications.
- The left arm is chosen so as not to miss a persistent left SVC with anomalous drainage to the left atrium.
- The stability of the image is checked during provocation maneuvers. These maneuvers are performed to transiently increase right atrial pressure and to provoke shunting through a potential interatrial communication.
- Typical maneuvers include a sharp nasal sniff, a cough, or the relaxation phase of the Valsalva maneuver.
- A positive test sees the rapid transit of bubbles from the right to the left heart within three to five cardiac cycles.
- The amount of bubbles seen is related to the size of the defect. Late transit (>5 cardiac cycles) of bubbles is associated with intrapulmonary shunting.

In addition to demonstrating the defect, TTE can demonstrate the hemodynamic consequences of the left to right shunt.

- Dilation of the right atrium and ventricle.
- Tricuspid valve annular dilation with associated tricuspid incompetence.
- Estimation of the peak right ventricular systolic pressure and in the absence of pulmonary valve stenosis an estimate of the systolic pulmonary artery pressure.

Associated lesions of the mitral valve (mitral valve prolapse, mitral stenosis), tricuspid valve (Ebstein's anomaly), and anomalous pulmonary venous drainage can also be looked for.

In the current era of percutaneous device closure of interatrial communications, transesophageal echocardiography (TEE) is mandatory prior to consideration of device closure. Many centers will do this immediately prior to a planned device closure. The key points regarding this are:

- Demonstration of all four pulmonary veins draining to the left atrium is essential prior to device closure of oval fossa defects.
- Ten per cent of secundum ASD have anomalous pulmonary venous drainage, most commonly of the right upper pulmonary vein.
- Exclude a superior sinus venosus defect, in the long axis 90 degree view and at zero degrees.
- Measure the margins of the atrial septum for suitability for device closure.
- A detailed mitral valve assessment is mandatory prior to closure as mitral incompetence is a potential complication of device closure.
- The severity of mitral stenosis and regurgitation are often underestimated in the presence of an ASD.
- Closure of a defect in the context of significant mitral valve disease will likely worsen symptoms, rather than improve them.
- Exclude intracardiac thrombus.

The roles of three-dimensional (3D) echocardiography and cardiac MRI have yet to be fully evaluated in the assessment of atrial septal defects, although both may have a role in defining non-invasively which patients are suitable for device closure of the defect.

Cardiac catheterization

Right heart catheterization is performed as part of the process of percutaneous device closure, via a femoral venous approach. Right and left heart catheterization is performed prior to planned surgery if the patient is older than 40 years, and/or coronary artery disease is suspected. If it is necessary to know the shunt size, this can be calculated by oximetry, with saturation sampling in the SVC, the IVC, the pulmonary artery, the pulmonary veins, and the femoral artery, using standard formulae to calculate the QP:QS.

CONCLUSIONS

Atrial septal defects often present in adult life but there is often a delay in the diagnosis being made. The symptoms are often mild or non-specific and the signs may be subtle. The use of routine investigations will enable the physician to accurately diagnose the presence of an atrial septal defect and plan the most appropriate management. This chapter summarizes the presenting features and relevant examination findings, and presents a guide to appropriate investigation and management of atrial septal defects in adults (Table 2.1).

Table 2.1 Summary of presenting features, examination findings, and investigations for small and large atrial communications

	Small atrial septal defect Defect <10 mm diameter QP:QS <1.5:1	Larger atrial septal defect QP:QS >1.5:1
Presenting features	Asymptomatic Routine examination Paradoxical embolus	Asymptomatic Routine examination Paradoxical embolus Effort intolerance Arrhythmia Heart failure
Examination	May be entirely normal	Pulmonary flow murmur Right ventricular heave Splitting of S2 Atrial arrhythmia

Investigations	Normal ECG
	Normal CXR
	ECHO atrial L-R shunt
	Catheter QP:QS <1.5:1
		ECG: RBBB, RAD, RVH
		CXR: enlarged heart & central
		  PAs with pulmonary plethora
		ECHO: volume loaded right
		  heart with atrial L-R shunt

Management	Leave if asymptomatic	Close in all cases

REFERENCES

1. Barber JM, Magidson O, Wood P. Atrial septal defect. Br Heart J 1950; 12(3):277–92.
2. Davia JE, Cheitlin MD, Bedynek JL. Sinus venosus atrial septal defect: analysis of fifty cases. Am Heart J 1973; 85(2):177–85.
3. Campbell M. Natural History of the atrial septal defect. Br Heart J 1970; 32:820–6.
4. Helber U, Baumann R, Sebolt H et al. Atrial septal defect in adults: cardiopulmonary exercise capacity before and 4 months and 10 years after defect closure. JACC 1997; 29:1345–50.
5. Gault JH, Morrow AG, Gay WA, Ross J. Atrial septal defects in patients over the age of forty years: clinical and hemodynamic studies and the effects of operation. Circulation 1968; 37:261–72.
6. Giardini A, Donti A, Formigari R et al. Determinants of cardiopulmonary functional improvement after transcatheter atrial septal defect closure in asymptomatic adults. JACC 2004; 43(10):1886–91.
7. Kobayashi Y, Nakanishi N, Kosakai Y. Pre- and postoperative exercise capacity associated with hemodynamics in adult patients with atrial septal defect: a retrospective study. Eur J Cardiothoracic Surgery 1997; 11:1062–6.
8. Jemielity M, Dyszkiewicz W, Paluszkiewicz L et al. Do patients over 40 years of age benefit from surgical closure of atrial septal defects? Heart 2001; 85(3):300–3.
9. Brochu MC, Baril JF, Dore A. Improvement in exercise capacity in asymptomatic and mildly symptomatic adults after atrial septal defect percutaneous closure. Circulation 2002; 106(14):1821–6.
10. Cowen ME, Jeffrey RR, Drakeley MJ et al. The results of surgery for atrial septal defect in patients aged fifty years and over. Eur Heart J 1990; 11(1):29–34.
11. Lechat P, Mas JL, Lascault G et al. Prevalence of patent foramen ovale in patients with stroke. New Engl J Med 1988; 318(18):1148–52.
12. Homma S, Sacco RL. Patent foramen ovale and stroke. Circulation 2005; 112:1063–72.

13. Morton JB, Sanders P, Vohra JK et al. Effect of chronic right atrial stretch on atrial electrical remodelling in patients with an atrial septal defect. Circulation 2003; 107:1175–782.
14. Murphy JG, Gersch BJ, McGoon MD et al. Long term outcome after surgical repair of isolated secundum atrial septal defect: follow up at 27–32 years. New Engl J Med 1990; 323:1645–50.
15. Silversides CK, Siu SC, McLaughlin PR et al. Symptomatic atrial arrhythmias and transcatheter closure of atrial septal defects in adult patients. Heart 2004; 90(10):1194–8.
16. Roos-Hesselink JW, Meijboom FJ, Spitaels SE et al. Excellent survival and low incidence of arrhythmias, stroke and heart failure long-term after surgical ASD closure at young age. A prospective follow-up study of 21–33 years. Eur Heart J 2003; 24(2):190–7.
17. Mantovan R, Gatzoulis MA, Pedrocco A et al. Supraventricular arrhythmia before and after surgical closure of atrial septal defects: spectrum, prognosis and management. Europace 2003; 5(2):133–8.
18. Gatzoulis MA, Freeman MA, Siu SC et al. Atrial arrhythmia after surgical closure of atrial septal defects in adults. New Engl J Med 1999; 340(11):839–46.
19. Sung RJ, Tamer DM, Agha AS et al. Etiology of the electrocardiographic pattern of "incomplete right bundle branch block" in atrial septal defect: an electrophysiologic study. J Pediatr 1975; 87(6 PT 2):1182–6.
20. Ruschhaupt DG, Khoury L, Thilenius OG. Electrophysiologic abnormalities of children with ostium secundum atrial septal defect. Am J Cardiol 1984; 53(11):1643–7.
21. Bolens M, Friedli B. Sinus node function and conduction system before and after surgery for secundum atrial septal defect: an electrophysiologic study. Am J Cardiol 1984; 53(10):1415–20.

3

The patent foramen ovale: clinical significance in cerebrovascular disease

Hugh S Markus

Etiology • Epidemiological studies determining the relative prevalence of PFO in stroke patients compared with controls • The risk of recurrent stroke in patients with PFO • Influence of treatment on natural history • Summary

ETIOLOGY

A patent foramen ovale (PFO) develops when fibrous adhesions fail to seal the atrial septum after birth, allowing the persistence of a potential shunt between the right and left atria of the heart. This is a common finding in the general population but the finding of increased incidence in patients with stroke, particularly those with cryptogenic stroke, has led to the suggestion that PFO may be a risk factor for stroke. This in turn has resulted in PFO closure being proposed as a treatment to prevent stroke. Whether this is an appropriate treatment can only be answered by large randomized trials which are in progress. However, there is already considerable data on the association between PFO and stroke which will be reviewed in this chapter. This will be considered under a number of headings:

1. Epidemiological studies determining the relative prevalence of PFO in stroke patients compared with controls.
2. The risk of recurrent stroke in patients with PFO.
3. Influence of treatment on recurrent stroke risk in patients with PFO
   a. Medical therapies.
   b. PFO closure.

A number of studies have also looked at the association between atrial septum aneurysm (ASA) and stroke, and these will also be covered in this review. Atrial septal aneurysm, originally described by Silver and Dorsey,[1] is defined as being present if the base of the aneurysmal protrusion measures ≤1.5 cm in diameter, and there is either a fixed protrusion of the fossa ovalis of at least 1–1.5 cm into an atrium or phasic excursion of the fossa ovalis throughout the cardiorespiratory cycle exceeding 1.5cm from the plane of the atrial septum.

EPIDEMIOLOGICAL STUDIES DETERMINING THE RELATIVE PREVALENCE OF PFO IN STROKE PATIENTS COMPARED WITH CONTROLS

Prevalence of PFO in the general population

An autopsy study of 965 normal hearts from patients with no history of cardioembolism found the prevalence of PFO present on probing to be 27%.[2] There was no difference in prevalence between men and women. A similar prevalence has been observed in an echocardiographic study, the Stroke Prevention Assessment of Risk in a Community (SPARC) Study.[3] A total of 588 healthy adult American residents <45 years of age were randomly selected and underwent transesophageal echocardiography (TEE) and carotid ultrasound to identify potential risk factors for stroke. PFO was found in 25.6% of individuals, and of those with PFO, the size was ≤1 mm in 46%, shunts were present at rest in 57%, and 92% had shunts after straining or coughing. The prevalence of ASA was much lower at 2.2%, although half of the subjects with ASA had concomitant PFO. Again the PFO prevalence was similar for men and women.

Association of PFO with stroke

The first report of paradoxical embolism as a potential stroke mechanism in a patient with PFO was by Cohnheim in 1877 during an autopsy study of a young woman. The most likely mechanism underlying this association is thought to be the passage of thrombus, or less commonly, other embolic material such as fat and air, from the venous side of the circulation to the left atrium via the PFO with subsequent passage to the brain. The most common source of venous embolism is deep venous thrombosis in the legs. Such paradoxical embolism can occur when right atrial pressure exceeds left atrial pressure. In patients with no underlying cardiopulmonary disease, mean left atrial pressure exceeds right atrial pressure. However, right atrial pressure may exceed left atrial pressure during normal inspiration, or after release of Valsalva maneuvers such as coughing and straining. There is no doubt that in some cases, paradoxical embolism through a PFO can cause stroke. Visualization of thrombus as it straddles the PFO on echocardiography is occasionally seen (Figure 3.1),[4] while in occasional postmortem cases an embolism passing through a PFO has been reported.[5,6] However, the important question is how common is this mechanism as a cause of stroke in patients with PFO? It is also important to remember that mechanisms other than paradoxical embolism could underlie any association between PFO and stroke. For example, thromboembolism could occur from the endocardial surface of the interatrial septum, or secondary to paroxysmal atrial fibrillation, or other arrhythmias associated with the PFO.[7–9]

To determine causality between PFO and stroke, it is necessary not only to demonstrate an association between the two, but also to demonstrate that removing the cause (that is, closing the PFO) results in a reduction in stroke risk. Many studies have examined epidemiological associations between PFO and stroke, but as yet there are only very limited data determining whether intervention can reduce stroke risk.

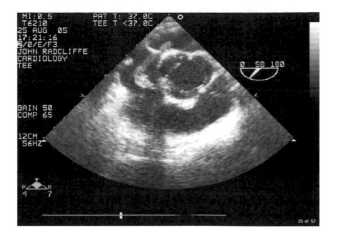

Figure 3.1a Transesophageal echocardiogram demonstrating thrombus traversing a patent foramen ovale

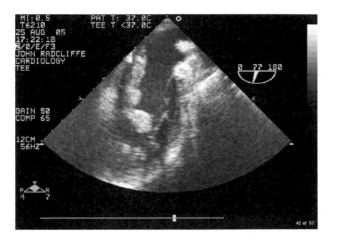

Figure 3.1b Transesophageal echocardiogram showing the same thrombus within the left ventricle

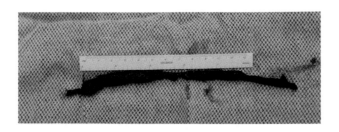

Figure 3.1c The thrombus when removed surgically

Figures 3.1a, 3.1b and 3.1c have been supplied by Dr. Oliver Ormerod, Consultant Cardiologist, John Radcliffe Hospital, Oxford, and we gratefully acknowledge his permission to reproduce them

Pathogenesis of stroke implications for interpreting an association

Before interpreting the data from studies investigating an association between PFO and stroke, it is helpful to understand the mechanisms of stroke in different patients. Stroke describes a syndrome of focal cerebral ischemia and is caused by a variety of different diseases with different disease mechanisms. About 20% is caused by primary cerebral hemorrhage, either intracerebral hemorrhage or subarachnoid hemorrhage. The remaining 80% is caused by ischemic stroke, and it is this subtype that has been associated with PFO. Approximately 20% of ischemic stroke is caused by large artery disease, usually atherosclerosis, and most commonly affecting the carotid and vertebral arteries. About a quarter of ischemic stroke is caused by small vessel disease of the perforating arteries resulting in lacunar infarction. The mechanisms of this stroke subtype are poorly understood. Hypertension is a major risk factor, while embolism appears to play a minor role. About a quarter of ischemic stroke is caused by cardioembolism. Important cardioembolic sources include atrial fibrillation, left ventricular akinetic segments, and poor function resulting in mural thrombus, valvular heart disease, and prosthetic cardiac valves. A small proportion of strokes are caused by other defined causes such as vasculitis, carotid and vertebral artery dissection, and rare genetic causes including sickle cell disease. Despite imaging of the brain, heart, and cerebral vessels, and appropriate investigations to look for specific causes, in about 25–40% of cases of ischemic stroke no cause can be found. This is called cryptogenic stroke. It is in this subgroup that associations with PFO have been most consistently reported. In older individuals atherosclerotic processes and atrial fibrillation become increasingly important in stroke pathogenesis, and it is probably for this reason that associations between PFO and stroke have been most consistent in younger individuals.

Case control studies associated PFO with stroke

A large number of case control studies have determined whether PFO is more common in patients with stroke compared with controls. Most of these have used echocardiography to detect PFO, although some more recent studies have used transcranial Doppler ultrasonography during agitated contrast injection. A systematic review and meta-analysis of these case control studies was published in 2000.[10] Data from 15 studies looking at PFO alone, 9 looking at ASA alone, and 4 looking at PFO plus ASA were analyzed. The odds ratio (OR) for PFO as a risk factor for stroke at any age was 1.83 (95%CI, 1.25–2.66). Significant heterogeneity was detected and this appeared to result largely from the different age of participants. If the trials were divided into two separate groups on the basis of positive studies, and neutral or negative studies, the mean age of patients in positive studies was found to be significantly lower than that in neutral or negative studies (44.8 years vs 61.8 years, $p = 0.022$). More homogeneous results were obtained from the nine studies in the younger age group, and the OR in individuals ≤55 years was 3.10 (95%CI, 2.29–4.21). In older individuals (≥55 years) more heterogeneous results were obtained and the odds ratio was not significant (1.27, 95%CI, 0.80–2.01).

The association between PFO and stroke appeared strongest in patients with young cryptogenic stroke. Twenty-two studies had looked at the incidence of PFO in cryptogenic stroke cases compared with stroke cases of known cause.

Although results were heterogeneous, an odds ratio of 3.16 (95%CI, 2.30–4.35) was found. Again heterogeneity was reduced in the younger age group, and in patients ≤55 years the odds ratio increased to 6.00 (95%CI, 3.72–9.68).

The meta-analysis also found a significant association between ASA and stroke with an OR of 2.35 (95%CI, 1.46–3.77) in all age groups, and this increased to 6.14 (95%CI, 2.47–15.22) when only studies of individuals ≤55 years were included. In patients 55 years or older, there was still a significant association with ASA, but this was weaker with an OR of 3.43 (95%CI, 1.89–6.22). As for PFO, ASA was found to be associated with cryptogenic stroke compared with strokes of known cause with an OR of 3.65 (95%CI, 1.34–9.97) with data from five studies.

Data from four studies were considered in evaluating the association between PFO plus ASA as a combined risk factor for stroke. The OR across all ages compared with normal controls was 4.96 (95%CI, 2.37–10.39) and increased to 15.59 (95%CI 2.83–85.87) for individuals ≤55 years. For older individuals the OR reduced to 5.09 (95%CI, 1.25–20.74). Only two studies compared prevalence rates in cryptogenic stroke compared with stroke of other known cause for PFO plus ASA; these revealed an odds ratio of 23.26 (95%CI, 5.24–103.20).

In any meta-analysis such as this, over-estimations may occur, not only due to publication bias, but also due to the differing methodologies used in different studies. The authors looked for publication bias by the use of funnel plots and only found slight evidence of this for some comparisons. Nevertheless, it cannot be completely excluded. However, this was a well performed meta-analysis and the results do provide convincing evidence that both PFO and ASA are more common in younger stroke patients compared with normal controls, and are more common in cryptogenic strokes compared with strokes of known cause. These findings would certainly be consistent with PFO and ASA being risk factors for stroke, but on their own they do not prove causality.

Indicators of increased risk from case control studies

A number of case control studies have attempted to identify clinical and echocardiographic markers of increased risk. Clinical features associated with increased risk in individual studies include a Valsalva maneuver preceding the stroke or TIA,[11] the presence of coexisting hypercoagulable or prothrombotic states,[12] and multiple strokes or TIAs.[11] Echocardiographic characteristics of the PFO associated with increased risk include large right-to-left shunting,[13,14] right-to-left shunting at rest,[15] and the presence of an ASA.[16–18]

THE RISK OF RECURRENT STROKE IN PATIENTS WITH PFO

An alternative approach is to prospectively follow patients with stroke and PFO/ASA to determine recurrent stroke rates. These can then be compared with patients with stroke due to other known causes. Such studies provide important information on the relative risk associated with PFO/ASA compared with other mechanisms of stroke, but they do not in themselves help decide whether PFO/ASA can cause stroke. It is also important to know the natural history and recurrence rate in patients with PFO and stroke to allow power calculations to be performed for intervention studies. A report from the American Academy of Neurology, published in 2004, carried out a systematic review of studies examining this association.[19] A large number of articles were reviewed but only four were considered to provide useful data. Two studies were graded as Class 1, one study as Class 2 and one study graded Class 4. The best data were obtained from the two Class 1 studies, the French PFO/ASA Study[20] and the Patent Foramen Ovale in Cryptogenic Stroke Study (PICSS).[21]

The French study prospectively followed 581 patients with cryptogenic stroke of <51 years of age (mean age 42.5 years). Of these, 216 (37%) had PFO, 10 (1.7%) had ASA and 51 (9%) had both. All patients were treated with aspirin 300 mg per day except for those patients who had a deep venous thrombosis or pulmonary embolism, who received oral anticoagulation with warfarin for 3–6 months. Investigators were not blinded to treatment but all outcomes were adjudicated by a blinded validation committee. Only two patients were lost to follow-up, and the mean duration of follow-up was 37.8 months. The average annual rate of subsequent stroke or death in PFO patients compared to non-PFO patients was 1.5% versus 1.8% (relative risk (RR) 0.9, 95%CI, 0.46–1.82). No relationship was found between PFO shunt size and recurrent stroke risk. Compared to patients without PFO, the RR associated with a small PFO shunt was 1.01 (95%CI, 0.23–4.52), and for a large shunt was 1.10 (95%CI, 0.39–3.11).

The PICSS[21] prospectively enrolled 630 stroke patients who were participating in the Warfarin-Aspirin Recurrent Stroke Study (WARSS). All patients in WARSS who had received a TEE as part of their evaluation, and also those who had a cryptogenic stroke and would agree to a TEE were eligible to participate. The average age was 59 years and a total of 312 (49%) were randomized to warfarin while 318 (50.5%) received aspirin. Both patients and physicians were blinded to the medication type. Of this cohort 265 (42%) had cryptogenic stroke and 365 (58%) had stroke of a known etiology. A PFO was found on TEE in 203 (33.8%), and an ASA in 69 (11.5%). The average annual risk of subsequent stroke or death was 7.4% among patients with PFO and 7.7% among those without PFO (RR=0.96, 95%CI, 0.64–1.44) in the entire study cohort. In the cryptogenic stroke subset of 265 patients, the average annual risk in the two groups was 7.15% and 6.35% respectively (RR=1.14, 95%CI, 0.60–2.17). Similar to the French study, there was no relationship between risk of recurrent stroke and PFO size. Compared to patients without PFO, the hazard ratio associated with a small PFO shunt was 1.23 (95%CI, 0.76–2.0) and for a large shunt was 0.59 (95%CI, 0.28–1.24).

Combining these two studies into a meta-analysis[19] revealed a pooled relative risk of recurrent stroke or death in PFO patients compared to non-PFO patients of 0.96 (95%CI, 0.59–1.55). Less robust data were obtained from a smaller study of 86 patients from Italy,[15] but addition of these data to the meta-analysis did not significantly alter the results.

The overall conclusion from these studies is that the presence of a PFO alone does not indicate an increased risk of recurrent stroke, although a small increase or decrease in risk cannot be excluded by the current data. However, this result does not prove or disprove an association between PFO and stroke. For example, in the non-PFO cases other definite causes have resulted in stroke in many cases. These also have a recurrent stroke risk. The above data have only demonstrated that the recurrent stroke risk is similar in patients with and without PFO.

The American Academy of Neurology Standard Sub-committee concluded that there were insufficient data in any of the studies to accurately estimate the relative risk associated with ASA alone.[19] In the French study,[20] 10 patients with lone ASA were included, none of whom reached an endpoint during the study period, while the PICSS did not provide data on patients who had an ASA exclusively.[21] In the French study there was a non-significant increase in risk in patients with both PFO and ASA compared to those without interatrial septal abnormalities (3.8% versus 1.8%, RR=2.10, 95%CI, 0.86–5.06). This difference became significant when stroke recurrence rate (not death) was included; RR=2.98, 95%CI, 1.17–7.58. In PICSS, amongst patients with any stroke subtype, the annual risk in patients with both PFO and ASA compared to those without any septal abnormality was not significantly elevated; 8.0% versus 7.7%, (RR=1.04, 95%CI 0.51–2.12). Data were not available for the subtype with cryptogenic stroke alone. Therefore firm conclusions are difficult to draw about the risk associated with PFO and ASA. An important difference between these two studies is that the mean age in the French study was 42.5 years and all patients were <51 years of age, while the mean age in PICSS was 59 years. This may be relevant to the differences in the studies, and could reflect an increased risk with PFO and ASA primarily in younger individuals.

INFLUENCE OF TREATMENT ON NATURAL HISTORY

Important evidence for causality could be provided by intervention studies with either medical, or particularly surgical procedures. Treatments used for secondary prevention in patients with stroke and PFO include anticoagulation, antiplatelet agents, and both surgical and more recently endovascular closure.

Medical therapies

It has been suggested that anticoagulation with warfarin may be more effective than antiplatelet agents such as aspirin, as secondary stroke prevention in patients with PFO and ASA and stroke. A meta-analysis of the limited data available published in 2001 reported a reduced risk with warfarin therapy.[22] However, most of the data available are from uncontrolled or unrandomized studies. The only randomized study is from the PICSS cohort.[21] A major strength of this study was that treatment was double blind, which entailed blood-taking for fictitious prothrombin time assays, even in patients treated with antiplatelet agents. This was an impressive undertaking. A limitation is that it was part of the larger WARSS randomized clinical trial, and therefore patients were randomized to this study rather than according to whether or not PFO and ASA were present. Nevertheless it does provide the most useful data (Figure 3.2). Among patients with any stroke subtype and PFO, there was no difference in the average annual rate of subsequent stroke or death between treatment with warfarin relative to aspirin (8.25% versus 6.6%, RR=1.25, 95%CI, 0.64–2.42). Among the cryptogenic cohort with PFO, there was again no difference between warfarin compared with aspirin-treated patients, although there was a marked trend towards a reduction in warfarin-treated patients (4.75% versus 8.95%, RR=0.53, 95%CI, 0.18–1.58). The wide confidence intervals make any firm conclusions impossible to draw, but the data would be consistent with benefit for warfarin therapy. Data from further randomized trials will be required to resolve this question. There were insufficient data from patients with both PFO and ASA to determine which therapy was most useful in this group.

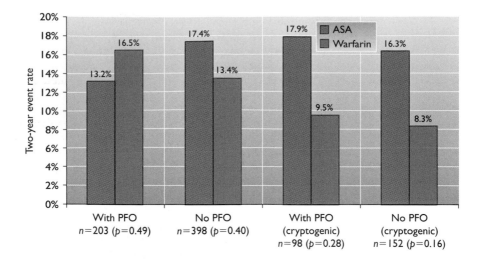

Figure 3.2 The risk of stroke in the PICSS study, according to treatment with aspirin (ASA) and warfarin. A non-significant reduction in two-year stroke or death rate can be seen in patients with PFO who are treated with warfarin. (Modified from reference 21.)

PFO closure

The most convincing evidence for causality of PFO in stroke pathogenesis would be if PFO closure resulted in an abolition of stroke recurrence risk. With the advent of relatively easy and low-risk closure of PFOs by percutaneous techniques, this hypothesis can now be tested. Currently there are no data available from randomized controlled trials to determine whether PFO closure does reduce stroke risk. However, a number of trials are currently under way such as the PC Trial using the Amplatzer® device, CLOSURE using the CardioSEAL® device, and RESPECT in the US using the Amplatzer® device. These are mostly examining the efficacy of closure in younger patients with cryptogenic stroke. Results will not be available for a number of years and the current planned studies are only moderately sized; larger studies may be required to obtain a definitive answer.

The only data currently available are from uncontrolled non-randomized studies. Extreme caution has to be used in interpreting these results for a number of reasons. Firstly, there may be significant publication bias with authors only publishing impressive results, and positive results being more easily accepted for publication. Secondly, the results are likely to be from pioneers in the area with particular expertise and may be less good when a technique is widely implemented in clinical practice. Nevertheless, they may provide useful pointers, particularly in how to plan larger-scale clinical studies.

Catheter closure of PFO was first reported in 1992 by Bridges and colleagues who used clam shell devices in 36 patients with presumed paradoxical events.[23] Following this, devices specifically designed for PFO closure were developed and the procedure has become widely available. Increasingly, numbers of reports of uncontrolled series have been published. A systematic review published in 2003 attempted to summarize the current status.[24] Outcome was compared in 10 studies of transcatheter closure involving 1,355 patients and six studies of medical therapy involving 895 patients. The one year rate of recurrent neurological thrombo-embolism with transcatheter intervention was 0–4.9%, with an incidence of major and minor complications of 1.5% and 7.9% respectively. Medical management was associated with a one year recurrence rate of 3.8–12%. However, great caution needs to be used in interpreting these results and any comparison between medical and interventional therapy is very diffi-cult. The medical studies involved older patients who had significantly more cardiovascular risk factors making direct comparison of recurrence rates impos-sible. Unfortunately, the systematic review did not identify which series were in patients with cryptogenic stroke in whom the association with PFO is much stronger as previously discussed, and which were in patients with PFO and other potential causes of stroke. Furthermore, no attempt was made to address the potentially great influence of publication bias. Since this meta-analysis, further larger studies have been published.[25-29] Again these are uncontrolled. Nevertheless, they do suggest that in younger patients with cryptogenic stroke who have their PFO closed, the risk of recurrent stroke is very low.

Before planning treatment trials in patients with PFO, it is important to have good estimates of the annual recurrent stroke risk to inform power calculations. A number of studies have addressed this issue and are listed in Table 3.1. In patients presenting with stroke and TIA who are found to have a PFO, and no other obvious cause for stroke, the annual recurrent stroke risk appears to be about 2% per year. The French PFO study reported a much higher risk in patients with PFO and ASA,[20] but this has not been replicated in other studies such as one in Bern, Switzerland which reported an annual stroke risk of 1.8% per annum.[30] The PICSS paper does not report recurrent stroke risk alone in patients with cryptogenic stroke.[21] There were 98 patients with cryptogenic stroke and PFO; annual recurrent stroke or death rates were 4.75% in the 42 warfarin-treated indi-viduals, and 8.95% in the 56 aspirin-treated individuals. These higher recurrence rates are likely to reflect not only the inclusion of death from causes other than stroke as an endpoint, but also the fact that the population was significantly older; therefore other causes of stroke such as atherosclerotic disease with a worse prognosis are likely to be important.

Table 3.1 The annual average risk of recurrent stroke, and stroke and TIA, in patients with PFO from prospective studies. (Adapted from reference 30)

Reference	Number of patients	Annual risk (%)	
		Stroke	Stroke and/or TIA
Mas[20]	132	1.2	3.4
Bogousslavsky[12]	140	2.4	3.8
De Castro[15]	74		2.4
Nedeltchev[30]	157	1.8	5.5

Therefore from available data it is reasonable to assume that the annual recurrent risk of stroke is 1–2% in younger patients with cryptogenic stroke and PFO. Data from closure studies in cryptogenic stroke suggest this can be reduced to between 0–2%. If one assumes that the rate in medically treated patients is 2% per year and this is reduced to 1.5% per annum (a 25% reduction) in patients treated with PFO closure, then a sample size of 14,178 with a follow-up of two years would be required to demonstrate a treatment effect. This would be reduced to 9,278 or 6,826 with follow-up extended to three and four years respectively. If the treatment effect was greater with a 50% stroke reduction from 2 to 1% per annum, the corresponding sample sizes would be 3,046, 1,986, and 1,472 with two, three and four years follow up respectively. These calculations assume a power of 0.9 and significance level of 0.05. They also assume no drop outs; in a real-life trail with drop-outs and treatment cross-overs, there would need to be an increase of perhaps 20%. As one can appreciate, these are large sample sizes and considerably larger than those planned for most of the current randomized controlled trials comparing PFO closure with medical treatment.

SUMMARY

There is considerable evidence supporting an association between PFO and ischemic stroke, particularly in individuals with cryptogenic stroke. This is consistent with a causal relationship, but does not prove causality. Non-randomized studies with PFO closure suggest the procedure may reduce recurrent stroke risk supporting a causal role for PFO in stroke pathogenesis, but firm conclusions are impossible to draw from these studies due to the potential bias inherent in such uncontrolled case series. Whether PFO closure really can prevent stroke can only be answered by randomized trials comparing closure with best medical therapy. Such trials are underway, but may be underpowered. Power calculations made using best available natural history data suggest that large sample sizes will be required.

REFERENCES

1. Silver MD, Dorsey JS. Aneurysms of the septum primum in adults. Arch Pathol Lab Med 1978; 102:62–5.
2. Hagen PT, Scholz DG, Edwards WD. Incidence and size of patent foramen ovale during the first 10 decades of life: an autopsy study of 965 normal hearts. Mayo Clin Proc 1984; 59:17–20.
3. Meissner I, Whisnant JP, Khandheria BK et al. Prevalence of potential risk factors for stroke assessed by transesophageal echocardiography and carotid ultrasonography: the SPARC study. Stroke Prevention: Assessment of Risk in a Community. Mayo Clin Proc 1999; 74:862–9.
4. Wu LA, Malouf JF, Dearani JA et al. Patent foramen ovale in cryptogenic stroke: current understanding and management options. Arch Intern Med 2004; 164:950–6.
5. Falk V, Walther T, Krankenberg H, Mohr FW. Trapped thrombus in a patent foramen ovale. Thorac Cardiovasc Surg 1997; 45:90–2.
6. Srivastava NT, Payment MF. Paradoxical embolism thrombus in transit through a patent foramen ovale. New Eng J Med 1997; 337:681.
7. Rice MJ, McDonald RW, Reller MD. Fetal atrial septal aneurysm: a cause of fetal atrial arrhythmias. J Am Coll Cardiol 1988; 12:1292–7.

8. Berthet K, Lavergne T, Cohen A et al. Significant association of atrial vulnerability with atrial septal abnormalities in young patients with ischemic stroke of unknown cause. Stroke 2000; 31:398–403.
9. Somody E, Albucher JF, Casteignau G et al. Anomalies of the interatrial septum and latent atrial vulnerability in unexplained ischemic stroke in young adults. Arch Mal Coeur Vaiss 2000; 93:1495–500.
10. Overell JR, Bone I, Lees KR. Interatrial septal abnormalities and stroke: a meta-analysis of case-control studies. Neurology 2000; 55:1172–9.
11. Dearani JA, Ugurlu BS, Danielson GK et al. Surgical patent foramen ovale closure for prevention of paradoxical embolism-related cerebrovascular ischemic events. Circulation 1999; 100 (suppl):II171–II175.
12. Bogousslavsky J, Garazi S, Jeanrenaud X, Aebischer N, Van Meile G, Lausanne Stroke with Paradoxical Embolism Study Group. Stroke recurrence in patients with patent foramen ovale: the Lausanne Study. Neurology 1996; 46:1301–5.
13. Homma S, Di Tullio MR, Sacco RL, Mihalatos D, Li Mandri G, Mohr JP. Characteristics of patent foramen ovale associated with cryptogenic stroke: a biplane transesophageal echocardiographic study. Stroke 1994; 25:582–6.
14. Stone DA, Godard J, Corretti MC et al. Patent foramen ovale: association between the degree of shunt by contrast transesophageal echocardiography and the risk of future ischemic neurologic events. Am Heart J 1996; 131:158–61.
15. De Castro S, Cartoni D, Fiorelli M et al. Morphological and functional characteristics of patent foramen ovale and their embolic implications. Stroke 2000; 31:2407–13.
16. Gallet B, Malergue MC, Adams C et al. Atrial septal aneurysm-a potential cause of systemic embolism: an echocardiographic study. Br Heart J 1985; 53:292–7.
17. Belkin RN, Hurwitz BJ, Kisslo J. Atrial septal aneurysm: association with cerebrovascular and peripheral embolic events. Stroke 1987; 18:856–62.
18. Hanna JP, Sun JP, Furlan AJ, Stewart WJ, Sila CA, Tan M. Patent foramen ovale and brain infarct: echocardiographic predictors, recurrence, and prevention. Stroke 1994; 25:782–6.
19. Messe SR, Silverman IE, Kizer JR et al. Quality Standards Subcommittee of the American Academy of Neurology. Practice parameter: recurrent stroke with patent foramen ovale and atrial septal aneurysm: report of the Quality Standards Subcommittee of the American Academy of Neurology. Neurology 2004; 62:1042–50.
20. Mas JL, Arquizan C, Lamy C et al. Recurrent cerebrovascular events associated with patent foramen ovale, atrial septal aneurysm, or both. New Engl J Med 2001; 345:1740–6.
21. Homma S, Sacco RL, Di Tullio MR, Sciacca RR, Mohr JP. Effect of medical treatment in stroke patients with patent foramen ovale: patent foramen ovale in cryptogenic stroke study. Circulation 2002; 105:2625–31.
22. Orgera MA, O'Malley PG, Taylor AJ. Secondary prevention of cerebral ischemia in patent foramen ovale: systematic review and meta-analysis. South Med J 2001; 94:699–703.
23. Bridges ND, Hellenbrand W, Latson L, Filiano J, Newburger JW, Lock JE. Transcatheter closure of patent foramen ovale after presumed paradoxical embolism. Circulation 1992; 86:1902–8.
24. Khairy P, O'Donnell CP, Landzberg MJ. Transcatheter closure versus medical therapy of patent foramen ovale and presumed paradoxical thromboemboli: a systematic review. Ann Intern Med 2003; 139:753–60.
25. Schuchlenz HW, Weihs W, Berghold A, Lechner A, Schmidt R. Secondary prevention after cryptogenic cerebrovascular events in patients with patent foramen ovale. Int J Cardiol 2005; 101:77–82.
26. Windecker S, Wahl A, Nedeltchev K et al. Comparison of medical treatment with percutaneous closure of patent foramen ovale in patients with cryptogenic stroke. J Am Coll Cardiol 2004; 44:750–8.
27. Braun M, Gliech V, Boscheri A et al. Transcatheter closure of patent foramen ovale (PFO) in patients with paradoxical embolism. Periprocedural safety and mid-term follow-up results of three different device occluder systems. Eur Heart J 2004; 25:424–30.

28. Khositseth A, Cabalka AK, Sweeney JP et al. Transcatheter Amplatzer device closure of atrial septal defect and patent foramen ovale in patients with presumed paradoxical embolism. Mayo Clin Proc 2004; 79:35–41.
29. Onorato E, Melzi G, Casilli F et al. Patent foramen ovale with paradoxical embolism: mid-term results of transcatheter closure in 256 patients. J Interv Cardiol 2003; 16:43–50.
30. Nedeltchev K, Arnold M, Wahl A et al. Outcome of patients with cryptogenic stroke and patent foramen ovale. J Neurol Neurosurg Psychiatry 2002; 72:347–50.

4

The patent foramen ovale: clinical significance in decompression illness and migraine

Peter Wilmshurst and Simon Nightingale

Introduction • Decompression illness • Sub-atmospheric decompression illness
• The link between decompression illness and migraine • Migraine

INTRODUCTION

The presence of a large patent (persistent) foramen ovale (PFO) is associated with an increased incidence of cryptogenic stroke (Chapter 3), some types of decompression illness,[1,2] migraine with aura,[3,4] and transient global amnesia.[5] Compared with the general population, people who experience migraine with aura have an increased risk of ischemic stroke,[6] decompression illness,[7] and transient global amnesia.[8] The increased risk of decompression illness in migraine sufferers is confined to those with a large PFO or another cause of large right-to-left shunt.[9] The inter-relationships of these diseases suggest that they share a common etiological mechanism, which is that large right-to-left shunts allow venous blood and its contents (including thrombo-emboli, gas bubbles, or chemical agents) to circumvent the pulmonary capillary bed and reach the systemic circulation. Although approximately a quarter of the population have a PFO, the clinical syndromes associated with a PFO are confined to those with the largest right-to-left shunts.

DECOMPRESSION ILLNESS

When ambient pressure is increased during a diver's descent under water, the increased partial pressure of nitrogen (or in certain situations other gases) in the diver's lungs produces an increase in the partial pressure of nitrogen in arterial blood and hence other tissues. As a result there is a proportionate increase in the amount of nitrogen dissolved in tissues. As the diver returns to the surface (during decompression), various tissues become supersaturated with nitrogen relative to the reduced ambient pressure, causing nitrogen bubble nucleation (Figure 4.1). In particular, bubbles form in venous blood.

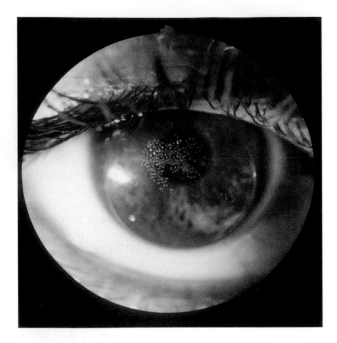

Figure 4.1 Bubbles formed in tear fluid beneath the contact lens of a diver during decompression.

The ambient pressure increases by one atmosphere (1 bar or 100 kPa) for every 10 m depth. At sea-level the tissues of an average-size adult contain several litres of highly fat-soluble nitrogen. If a diver descends to 30 m, where the ambient pressure is 4 bar, tissue nitrogen content will gradually increase until at equilibrium the tissues will contain four times as many nitrogen molecules as were dissolved at the surface. The rate of ascent (decompression) should be slow, such that the rate of bubble nucleation in venous blood and other tissues is low.

It is common for a few nitrogen bubbles to form in venous blood following innocuous dives. Usually the bubbles collapse during passage through the alveolar capillaries as nitrogen passes down the concentration gradient into the alveoli, so that bubbles do not pass into the systemic circulation. However, when the dive profile is provocative, because of a large uptake of nitrogen during a deep and long dive and because decompression was rapid, the massive amounts of bubbles nucleated in venous blood may overwhelm the pulmonary filter, so that bubbles reach the systemic circulation to embolize critical tissues.[10] These tissues are also supersaturated with nitrogen so that bubble emboli are amplified as nitrogen passes down the concentration gradient from the supersaturated tissues into the bubbles. Expanding bubble emboli in critical tissues, particularly the central nervous system, cause decompression illness. Bubble amplification does not happen in contrast echocardiography when there is a right-to-left shunt, because in that situation the bubbles' emboli enter tissues that are not supersaturated with dissolved inert gas. Therefore, the bubbles' do not expand, but will collapse because the pressure gradient is from bubble to tissue.

Decompression illness can also occur when systemic arterial gas embolism occurs by a different mechanism. If gas trapping as a result of lung disease or failure to exhale adequately during ascent (usually a rapid or emergency ascent) causes pulmonary barotrauma, bubbles may invade the pulmonary veins to become arterial gas emboli. At the time of gas embolism during ascent, all tissues are supersaturated with nitrogen so the effects are greatest in critical tissues with high blood flow, and it causes predominantly cerebral or cardiac effects.

However, most episodes of decompression illness cannot be explained by these mechanisms, since the dive profile was not provocative and the diver did not have lung disease. An explanation was proposed in 1986, when a man with an atrial septal defect had decompression illness after a theoretically safe dive that should have caused only a small amount of venous gas nucleation.[11] It was proposed that even when there is relatively little venous bubble formation during decompression, a right-to-left shunt may allow paradoxical gas embolism. In this way the venous bubbles evade the pulmonary filter and pass into the systemic circulation to embolize critical tissues and cause decompression illness.[11]

In 1989, Moon and colleagues reported that 11 of 18 (61%) patients with a history of serious neurological decompression illness had a right-to-left shunt consistent with the presence of a PFO on transthoracic contrast echocardiography compared with a shunt rate of 9 in 176 (5%) of historic controls ($p = 0.0001$).[1] Another case controlled study showed that neurological decompression illness, following a non-provocative dive, usually occurred in divers who had a shunt, whereas after a provocative dive, the divers usually had no shunt.[2,12,13] Neurological symptoms with latency (time to onset) within 30 minutes of surfacing, as well as cutaneous and cardio-respiratory decompression illness were strongly associated with the presence of a right-to-left shunt, but that joint pain was not.[2,12,13] Because, at the time, these findings were controversial, a replication study was performed under supervision of staff of the Medical Research Council and members of the MRC Decompression Sickness Panel and confirmed these findings.[14] Since then many studies in divers with decompression illness have provided more information about the types of decompression illness associated with shunts and the type and size of shunts responsible.

Results

A blind case control study to determine the relationship between different manifestations of neurological decompression illness and its causes in 100 consecutive divers with neurological decompression illness and 123 historical control divers, found that the size of right-to-left shunts was critical to development of decompression illness.[15] A large shunt was seen after a single injection of bubble contrast at rest in 41 of 100 (41%) cases compared with 6 of 123 (4.9%) of controls ($p < 0.001$). A Valsalva maneuver increased the rates of large shunts detected to 51% of cases and 7.3% of controls ($p < 0.001$). Shunts graded large or medium in size were present in 52% of affected divers and 12.2% of controls ($p < 0.001$). Spinal decompression illness occurred in 26 of 52 affected divers with large or medium size shunts and in 12 of 48 without ($p < 0.02$). The distribution of latencies of decompression illness symptoms differed markedly between the 52 divers with a large or medium shunt, and the 30 divers who had lung disease or a provocative dive profile. These studies have provided data that allow the cause of neurological decompression illness to be determined in most cases by taking a history of the dive profile and latency of onset, and by performing investigations to detect a right-to-left shunt or lung disease.

Since then other studies have consistently confirmed that right-to-left shunting across a PFO and, in particular, a large shunt is strongly associated with cerebral and cochleovestibular decompression illness.[16,17] The issue of whether spinal decompression illness is also shunt related is more controversial. All studies have found a significant relationship between spinal decompression illness and shunts,[2,15,17,18] with the exception of one small study,[16] of 20 cases of cerebral decompression illness compared with 20 controls, and 17 cases of spinal decompression illness compared with 16 controls. Unfortunately the rates of PFOs were very different in the two control groups (25% in the controls for cerebral cases and 50% in controls for spinal cases). With the exception of this poorly controlled study, the data suggest that spinal decompression illness is also strongly associated with a shunt.

If decompression illness is usually due to systemic arterial gas emboli, it is surprising that spinal decompression illness is so common, as the blood flow to the cord is much less than to the brain. This propensity for spinal manifestations in shunt-related decompression illness can be explained by the observation that after decompression there is an interval of a few minutes before bubbles are detected in venous blood. Bubbles crossing a shunt will pass to tissues with the greatest blood flow, such as the brain. However, the short nitrogen elimination half-life of the brain is such that by the time most bubbles reach it, it contains little dissolved nitrogen to amplify embolic bubbles. Far fewer bubble emboli enter the spinal cord, but they do so at a time when the cord, with its longer nitrogen elimination half-life, is still supersaturated and able to amplify bubble emboli. This hypothesis is supported by studies of the latency of onset of neurological symptoms in divers with a shunt,[15] and by observations of appearance times of bubbles in pulmonary arteries and in the arterial circulation in pigs with and without a PFO.[10]

The central role of right-to-left shunts in decompression illness is supported by studies on cutaneous decompression illness.[2,13,19] Few people expected that the rash of cutaneous decompression illness (Figure 4.2) could be the result of embolism. A small number of studies demonstrate that cutaneous decompression illness is also usually associated with a right-to-left shunt, though an embolic etiology of a diffuse rash is more difficult to explain.[2,13,19] A retrospective case control comparison of the prevalence and sizes of right-to-left shunts determined by contrast echocardiography performed blind to history in 61 divers (including one caisson worker) with a history of cutaneous decompression illness and 123 historical control divers found that 47 of the 61 (77%) cases with cutaneous decompression illness had a shunt compared with 34 of 123 (27.6%) control divers ($p < 0.001$).[19] The size of the shunts in those with cutaneous decompression illness was significantly larger than in the controls. Of 61 cases with cutaneous decompression illness, 30 (49.2%) had a large shunt at rest compared with 6 of 123 (4.9%) controls ($p < 0.001$). During closure procedures in 17 divers who had cutaneous decompression illness the mean diameter of foramen ovale was 10.9 mm. Cutaneous decompression illness occurred after dives that were provocative in those without shunts and after shallower and non-provocative dives in those with shunts. Those with shunts were also at increased risk of neurological decompression illness. These findings strongly

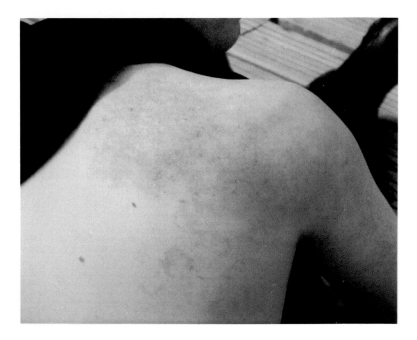

Figure 4.2   The mottled or 'marbled' rash of cutaneous decompression illness.

support the hypothesis that cutaneous decompression illness is usually due to paradoxical gas embolism with peripheral amplification in skin and subcutaneous fat supersaturated with nitrogen. Cutaneous decompression illness in those without a shunt also will occur if the lung filter is overwhelmed by venous bubbles or if there is autochthonous bubble formation (bubble nucleation in the skin rather than embolization of bubbles).[19]

Transcatheter closure of atrial shunts to prevent recurrence of decompression illness in divers was first reported in 1996.[20] Initially the procedure was restricted to commercial divers, for whom inability to return to unrestricted diving had serious financial consequences. At that stage amateur divers were advised to stop diving or to perform restricted diving so that the uptake of nitrogen was minimized with a reduced risk of venous bubble nucleation during decompression. If bubbles did form and cross the shunt, the modest nitrogen load in tissues would not produce much bubble amplification. Restricted diving or abstinence are options, but increasingly amateur divers who have had shunt-related decompression illness request PFO closure to permit unrestricted diving.[21,22] We have referred over 200 divers with a history of shunt-related decompression illness for transcatheter closure to date. At the time of PFO closure, the median diameter of defects was 11 mm.[22]

Before referring a diver for transcatheter closure of a PFO, we recommend that all four of the following criteria are satisfied:

1. There is no other cause for decompression illness. For example, provocative dive profile and lung disease that could cause gas trapping should be excluded.
2. The dive profile would have liberated some venous bubbles. This can be determined from dive tables.
3. The symptoms are consistent with shunt-related decompression illness. These include cutaneous decompression illness after a dive shallower than 50 m, • cardio-respiratory symptoms or neurological symptoms starting within 30 minutes of surfacing, migraine aura after surfacing, or a combination of these symptoms. The presence of joint pain suggests that the decompression illness was not shunt-related, except when pain is experienced in a joint over which there is the characteristic rash of cutaneous decompression illness.
4. Investigation demonstrates a significant right-to-left shunt with features consistent with an atrial defect.

Before return to diving after PFO closure, contrast echocardiography should confirm that there is no significant residual shunt.

SUB-ATMOSPHERIC DECOMPRESSION ILLNESS

Decompression illness can also occur during sub-atmospheric decompression in high-altitude aviators and in astronauts on space walks. Human terrestrial hypobaric chamber experiments indicate that gas nucleation occurs in body tissues with all decompression protocols studied.[23] Monitoring the pulmonary artery with Doppler ultrasound reveals that heavy burdens of circulating gaseous emboli are present in from 6 to 39% of those subjected to subatmospheric decompression.[23] In these hypobaric chamber studies serious decompression illness has been encountered, including massive cutaneous 'marbling' (characteristic of cutaneous decompression illness), severe cerebral dysfunction and circulatory shock.[24] A PFO screen was performed by the National Aeronautics and Space Administration (NASA) after four cases of serious decompression illness resulted from space-walk simulations. Contrast transthoracic echocardiography detected a PFO at rest in three.[23]

THE LINK BETWEEN DECOMPRESSION ILLNESS AND MIGRAINE

It has been recognized for 60 years that individuals who have migraine with aura have an increased risk of decompression illness and often experience migraine symptoms, particularly migraine visual aura, during sub-atmospheric decompression.[7] Divers who have migraine with aura (always visual aura but sometimes also hemiplegic, hemisensory, dysphasic or cognitive features) also often experience an identical migraine aura with or without headache following dives.[9] This only occurs in divers who have a clinically significant right-to-left shunt (usually a large PFO, but sometimes a pulmonary shunt) following dives that liberate venous bubbles.[9] In some the same migraine aura is experienced after right-to-left shunting of bubbles during contrast echocardiography.[9] The association between a history of migraine with aura and the increased risk of decompression illness is because migraine with aura is an indicator of an increased prevalence of large right-to-left shunts.

MIGRAINE

Recurrent migraine affects about 7% of men and 20% of women between ages 20 and 64.[25] In 1999 the economic burden of migraine in the USA from lost days of work, reduced productivity and medical treatment costs was estimated to be $14,574 million.[25] The figures used to calculate these costs were in line with those in Britain so that the equivalent figures for the UK population would have been £1,913 million, which was equivalent to 1p on the standard rate of income tax or about 0.5% of Gross Domestic Product.[26]

Using transcranial Doppler, right-to-left shunts that were presumed to be across PFOs were found in 41% of patients with migraine with aura, versus 16% of controls ($p < 0.005$) in one study,[3] and in 48% of patients with migraine with aura versus 20% of controls ($p < 0.01$) in another study.[4] The prevalence of shunts did not differ significantly between patients who had migraine without aura and controls.[4]

In a study of 400 divers who had contrast echocardiography following decompression illness, there was a relationship between size of right-to-left shunts and prevalence of migraine with aura (Table 4.1).[27] A large shunt at rest was present in 170 (42.5%), 33 (8.25%) had a large shunt with a Valsalva maneuver, 12 (3%) had a medium shunt, 24 (6%) had a small shunt and 161 (40.25%) had no shunt. Small shunts are not considered to have clinical significance; in those divers and those with no shunt, decompression illness was believed to be the result of a provocative dive profile or pulmonary barotrauma as a result of lung disease. In those with no shunt or only a small shunt, the lifetime prevalence of migraine with aura was similar to the general population (11%). Ninety of the 170 with large shunts at rest (53%) had migraine with aura. In those with large shunts with a Valsalva maneuver or a medium shunt, the lifetime prevalence of migraine with aura was intermediate at 21% and 25% respectively.

Genetic factors

A family history is present in up to 90% of patients with migraine and usually there is dominant inheritance with incomplete penetrance.[28] Atrial shunts (large

Table 4.1 The relationship between size of right-to-left shunt and prevalence of migraine with aura in divers with decompression illness[27]

Size of shunt	No. of divers with decompression illness	No. with migraine with aura	% with migraine with aura
No shunt	161	19	12
Small shunt	24	1	4
Medium shunt	12	3	25
Large shunt with a Valsalva maneuver	33	7	21
Large shunt at rest	170	90	53

PFOs or atrial septal defects) are also dominantly inherited in many families.[29] In some families, inheritance of migraine is closely linked to inheritance of atrial shunts.[29] In the families reported there was also a high prevalence of other shunt-related events. For example, in the family shown in the pedigree (Figure 4.3) the proband had episodes of shunt-related neurologic and cutaneous decompression illness. She had migraine aura at the times of her decompression illness and after other dives. She also had a 25-year history of migraine with aura unrelated to diving. She had transcatheter closure of a 10 mm diameter PFO and a 4 mm diameter atrial septal defect. Her sister, nephew, and mother had migraine with aura and each had a large right-to-left shunt with characteristics of a large PFO. Her mother also had a history of stroke at the age of 30 years and transient global amnesia.

The association between inheritance of PFOs and atrial septal defects and inheritance of migraine with aura is unlikely to be the result of co-segregation of genes situated close together on the same chromosome, but appears to be a causal association for two reasons. Firstly, right-to-left pulmonary shunts are also associated with migraine with aura.[9,27] In migraine with aura or migraine aura without headache pulmonary shunts are considerably more frequent than expected by chance.[30,31] In one study 50% of patients with hereditary hemorrhagic

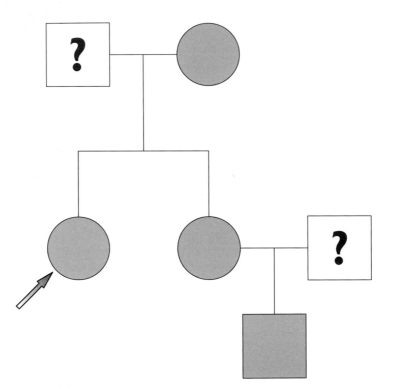

Figure 4.3 The pedigree of a family in which there is inheritance of both migraine with aura and an atrial shunt, represented by shaded symbols. The proband had shunt-related decompression illness. Her mother had stroke at age 30 years and transient global amnesia.

telangiectasia had migraine with aura and a further 3% had aura without headache.[32] This prevalence was four times greater than in the control group with another inherited condition, familial adenomatous polyposis, and 10 times greater than expected in population studies. The association between migraine with aura and hereditary hemorrhagic telangiectasia is unlikely to be the result of cerebral arteriovenous malformations, because these are found on MRI scans in only 6–8%, whereas pulmonary arteriovenous malformations are much commoner.[33]

Secondly there is increasing evidence that transcatheter closure of a PFO improves migraine. Transcatheter closure of large PFOs is performed when patients have had ischemic stroke that is believed to be the result of paradoxical thrombo-embolism or have had decompression illness that is believed to be the result of paradoxical gas embolism. In the first report to describe the effect of PFO closure for these indications, a consultant neurologist, who was blind to information about residual shunt, conducted a structured interview with individuals who had had percutaneous transcatheter closure of an atrial septal defect or PFO to determine how the procedure affected migraine symptoms.[34] Of 40 consecutive patients who had a closure procedure, 37 could be contacted, of whom 21 (56.8%) had a history of migraine prior to the procedure. Of these 21 cases, 16 (43.2%) had migraine with aura and five (13.5%) had migraine without aura. In the immediate post-closure period, 11 patients had visual aura. This period was disregarded for the long-term assessment. During long-term follow-up no migraine symptoms were reported by seven patients who had experienced migraine with aura preclosure and three who had experienced migraine without aura preclosure. In addition, eight others who had experienced migraine with aura preclosure reported improvement in frequency and severity of migraines. Only one who had experienced migraine with aura preclosure and two with migraine without aura preclosure reported no alteration in migraine episodes. It is unlikely that the improvement in migraine symptoms was the result of a placebo effect because the patients had no prior expectation that the procedure would improve their migraine. These observations suggest a causal association between right-to-left shunts and migraine with aura.

Since then, other groups have reported broadly similar results (Table 4.2).[35–40] All studies have found that the patients presenting with presumed paradoxical

Table 4.2 Papers reporting the effect of PFO closure on migraine

Study	No. of patients with PFO closed	No. with migraine	% with migraine	% with migraine improved or cured	Length of follow up (months)
Wilmshurst et al[34]	37	21	57	86	up to 30
Morandi et al[35]	62	17	27	88	all 6
Schwerzmann et al[36]	215	48	22	81	all 12
Post et al[37]	66	26	39	65 free from migraine	all 6
Reisman et al[38]	120	50	42	90	mean 4
Azarbal et al[39]	89	37	42	76	all 3
Reisman et al[40]	162	57	35	70	all 12

embolism and a large PFO have a higher prevalence of migraine than is found in population studies. (Some studies do not distinguish between migraine with aura and migraine without aura.) All studies report an improvement in migraine symptoms in many patients, and in many cases there is no recurrence of migraine. Overall the studies report that about 80% of patients find that they are either free from migraine or it is improved after transcatheter closure of their PFO.

However, it is clear that there is no absolute association between right-to-left shunts and migraine with aura. Some people with migraine have no shunt and some people with large shunts have no migraine. Even closure of a large PFO in someone with migraine does not have a predictable effect on migraine symptoms: some have no more migraine, some have less frequent or less severe migraine, some are unchanged. For some, migraine is worse particularly in the early weeks after the procedure.

How can these observations be reconciled? We postulated that migraine has a number of causes with similarities to the causes of decompression illness. In some people with migraine, venous blood contains one or more substances that can trigger an attack of migraine if it reaches the brain in sufficient concentrations.[9,34] These potential trigger substances in venous blood are normally filtered in the lungs where emboli are trapped and lung enzymes destroy many chemicals. A right-to-left shunt could permit trigger substances to circumvent the lung filter, which would increase the frequency or severity of migraine attacks in those individuals susceptible to the trigger substance. This is analogous to paradoxical gas embolism in divers with a large shunt, in whom venous bubbles circumvent the lung filter to reach the brain, which is susceptible to bubble emboli because it is supersaturated with nitrogen. In these migraine patients, closing the shunt would raise the threshold, so that some individuals have fewer or milder attacks and some have no more attacks.

However there will be individuals without a shunt who will experience attacks of migraine with aura, if their lung filter were less efficient, if the amount of trigger substance in venous blood were to overwhelm the lung filter, if their particular triggers were unaffected by transit through the lungs, or if the final common neural mechanism producing migraine were particularly sensitive to the trigger. This is analogous to a provocative dive that produces so many venous bubbles that the diver's lung filter is overwhelmed, allowing bubbles into the systemic arteries.

What might the trigger substance be? Migraine with aura and aura alone can occur in divers following decompression if the dive liberates venous bubbles, and if the diver has a large shunt.[9] These individuals sometimes also get migraine with aura following contrast echocardiography when many bubbles are seen to cross the atrial septum.[9] This does not occur in individuals with no shunt. Although an embolic mechanism is possible, it seems more probable that bubble emboli trigger migraine because platelets adhere to and become activated by bubbles.[9] Platelet activation liberates 5-HT. However venous 5-HT is virtually completely eliminated on passage through the lungs probably by alveolar monoamine oxidase.[41] Various observations suggest a role for 5-HT in migraine pathogenesis.[42] Antagonists of 5-HT receptors are commonly used to treat migraine.[42] There is also evidence that aspirin, a weak anti-platelet drug, reduces migraine.[43]

Some individuals notice that their migraines increase for a few weeks after transcatheter closure of a PFO.[34] In most cases this exacerbation abates after a few weeks, at a time when the occlusion device has been covered by endothelium. Prior to endothelialization the occlusion device is a potent platelet activator. Platelets activated on the left atrial part of the occlusion device will release 5-HT beyond the lung filter. This situation is analogous to decompression illness caused by bubble invasion of the pulmonary veins as a result of pulmonary barotrauma. A number of observations support platelet activation in the left heart as a possible etiological mechanism in some patients with migraine. For example, some patients get migraine symptoms for the first time after they have replacement of left heart valves with mechanical prosthetic valves (unpublished observations). Migraine is also associated with mitral leaflet prolapse.[44] Disappearance of migraine following removal of left atrial myxomas is described.[45] In addition, the early exacerbation of migraine with aura after transcatheter PFO closure can be prevented by treatment with the potent anti-platelet drug, clopidogrel.[46,47]

Definitive evidence for the role of large PFOs in the etiology of migraine with aura was sought in the MIST (Migraine Intervention with STARFlex® Technology) Trial. This multicenter study used a randomized double-blind comparison of transcatheter closure of PFO against sham intervention to determine whether previous reports of migraine relief following PFO closure were purely a placebo effect. The trial recruited patients with frequent attacks of migraine (at least five days of migraine per month), who had some migraine aura and who had failed to respond to at least two classes of prophylactic medications. They had cardiac assessment to exclude the presence of coincidental cardiac disease. If transthoracic contrast echocardiography showed a significant atrial right-to-left shunt consistent with the presence of a large PFO, they were eligible for randomization under general anesthetic to transcatheter closure of the PFO with a STARFlex® implant or sham intervention. Balloon sizing of the defect was performed during the closure procedure. Follow-up was by headache specialists who, like the patients, were blind to randomization assignment. Those patients who had implant procedures had repeat contrast echocardiography at the end of the study to determine whether there was a residual shunt.

Preliminary results from the MIST Trial were presented at the Late Breaking Clinical Trials Sessions of the i2 Summit at the Scientific Sessions of the American College of Cardiology in March 2006. The transthoracic contrast echocardiography results of the 432 patients with migraine enrolled in the MIST Trial are shown in Table 4.3. The three patients with atrial septal defects had evidence of right heart dilatation. They were not randomized but went on to defect closure outside the study. Of the 163 with significant shunts in keeping with a large PFO on contrast echocardiography, 16 either withdrew consent or were withdrawn for medical reasons before randomization. The remaining 147 were randomized with 74 having transcatheter closure and 73 having a sham intervention. The mean PFO diameter (±standard deviation) in those who had transcatheter closure was 9.2±3.3 mm.[31] These sizes are comparable to diameters of PFOs found in divers with PFO-related decompression illness.[22]

Preliminary analysis of the headache data shows that the primary end-point of elimination of headache was not achieved in this group of migraine patients who had severe, frequent, and refractory migraine. Such a difficult primary endpoint has never been sought in any other migraine study. The most

Table 4.3   The size and types of right-to-left shunts in patients with migraine in the MIST study[31]

	Number of patients	% of total number of patients
Total who had contrast echocardiography	432	100
Small shunts (atrial and pulmonary)	72	16.7
Large pulmonary shunts	22	5.1
Atrial septal defects	3	0.7
Large PFO	163	37.7
All large right-to-left shunts	188	43.5
All right-to-left shunts	260	60.2

commonly used endpoint used in migraine prophylaxis studies is the number of patients achieving a 50% reduction in days of migraine headaches. In the MIST study, significantly more patients with an implant than those who had the sham procedure had a 50% reduction of migraine headache days (42% v 23%, $p = 0.038$). Headache burden (frequency × duration of migraine headaches) was also reduced significantly more in those with an implant than in those with the sham intervention (37% v 17%, $p = 0.033$). The response observed in the sham group was comparable to the effects observed in placebo groups in drug trials of migraine prophylaxis. This confirms the necessity for proper sham groups in migraine intervention trials.

Further analysis of the MIST Trial is in progress, particularly to determine whether patients had residual shunting at the end of the study and how that affected outcomes, but it is apparent that transcatheter closure of PFO with the STARFlex® implant does improve migraine in some patients. Further research is in progress to determine whether the benefit is maintained long term and to determine which sub-groups obtain greatest benefit from the procedure.

References

1. Moon RE, Camporesi EM, Kisslo JA. Patent foramen and decompression sickness in divers. Lancet 1989; i:513–14.
2. Wilmshurst PT, Byrne JC, Webb-Peploe MM. Relation between interatrial shunts and decompression sickness in divers. Lancet 1989; ii:1302–6.
3. Del Sette M, Angeli S, Leandri M et al. Migraine with aura and right-to-left shunt on transcranial doppler: a case-control study. Cerebrovasc Dis 1998; 8:327–30.
4. Anzola GP, Magoni M, Guindani M, Rozzini L, Dalla Volta G. Potential source of cerebral embolism in migraine with aura. A transcranial doppler study. Neurology 1999; 52:1622–5.
5. Klotzsch C, Sliwka U, Berlit P, Noth J. An increased frequency of patent foramen ovale in patients with transient global amnesia. Analysis of 53 consecutive patients. Arch Neurol 1996:53:504–8.
6. Etminan M, Takkoucke B, Isorna FC, Samii A. Risk of ischaemic stroke in people with migraine: systematic review and meta-analysis of observational studies. BMJ 2005; 330:63–5.
7. Engel GL, Webb JP, Ferris EB, Romano J, Ryder H, Blankenhorn MA. A migraine-like syndrome complicating decompression sickness. War Medicine 1944; 5:304–14.
8. Caplan L, Chedru F, Lhermitte F, Mayman C. Transient global amnesia and migraine. Neurology 1981; 31:1167–70.

9. Wilmshurst P, Nightingale S. Relationship between migraine and cardiac and pulmonary right-to-left shunts. Clin Sci 2001; 100:215–20.

10. Vik A, Jenssen BM, Brubbakk AO. Arterial gas bubbles after decompression in pigs with patent foramen ovale. Undersea Biomed Res 1993; 20:121–31.

11. Wilmshurst PT, Ellis BG, Jenkins BS. Paradoxical gas embolism in a scuba diver with an atrial septal defect. BMJ 1986; 293:1277.

12. Wilmshurst PT, Byrne JC, Webb-Peploe MM. Neurological decompression sickness. Lancet 1989; i:731.

13. Wilmshurst PT, Byrne JC, Webb-Peploe MM. Relation between interatrial shunts and decompression sickness in divers. In: Sterk W, Geeraedts L, eds. EUBS 1990 Proceedings, London. European Undersea Biomedical Society 1990; 147–53.

14. Wilmshurst P. Interatrial shunts and decompression sickness in divers. Lancet 1990; 335:915.

15. Wilmshurst P, Bryson P. Relationship between the clinical features of neurological decompression illness and its causes. Clin Sci 2000; 99:65–75.

16. Germonpre P, Dendale P, Unger P, Balestra C. Patent foramen ovale and decompression sickness in sport divers. J Appl Physiol 1998; 84:1622–6.

17. Cantais E, Louge P, Suppini A, Foster P, Palmier B. Right-to-left shunt and risk of decompression illness with cochleovestibular and cerebral symptoms in divers: case control study in 101 consecutive dive accidents. Crit Care Med 2003; 31: 84–8.

18. Wilmshurst P, Davidson C, O'Connell G, Byrne C. Role of cardiorespiratory abnormalities, smoking and dive characteristics in the manifestations of neurological decompression illness. Clin Sci 1994; 86:297–303.

19. Wilmshurst PT, Pearson MJ, Walsh KP, Morrison WL. Relationship between right-to-left shunts and cutaneous decompression illness. Clin Sci 2001; 100:539–42.

20. Wilmshurst P, Walsh K, Morrison L. Transcatheter occlusion of foramen ovale with a button device after neurological decompression illness in professional divers. Lancet 1996; 348:752–3.

21. Walsh KP, Wilmshurst PT, Morrison WL. Transcatheter closure of patent foramen ovale using the Amplatzer septal occluder to prevent recurrence of neurological decompression illness in divers. Heart 1999; 257–61.

22. Wilmshurst P. Foramen ovale permeable et plongee: quelle strategie? In: Brion R, Coeur et Plongee, Paris. Published Communication Globale Sante, 2003; 33–9.

23. Kerut EK, Norfleet WT, Plotnick GD, Giles TD. Patent foramen ovale: a review of associated conditions and impact of physiological size. J Am Coll Cardiol 2001; 38:613–23.

24. Powell MR, Norfleet WT, Kumar KV, Butler BD. Patent foramen ovale and hypobaric decompression. Aviat Space Environ Med 1995; 66:273–5.

25. Hu XH, Markson LE, Lipton RB, Steward WF, Berger ML. Burden of migraine in the United States: disability and economic costs. Arch Intern Med 1999; 159:813–18.

26. Anonymous. Migraine: costs and consequences. Bandolier 1999; 67:5–6.

27. Wilmshurst P, Pearson M, Nightingale S. Re-evaluation of the relationship between migraine and persistent foramen ovale and other right-to-left shunts. Clin Sci 2005; 108:365–76.

28. Bradley WG, Daroff RB, Fenichel GM, Marsden CD. Neurology in clinical practice. Third edition. London, Butterworth-Heineman 2000; 1846.

29. Wilmshurst PT, Pearson MJ, Nightingale S, Walsh KP, Morrison WL. Inheritance of persistent foramen ovale and atrial septal defects and the relationship to familial migraine with aura. Heart 2004; 90:1315–20.

30. Wilmshurst P, Dowson A, Mullen M, Muir K, Nightingale S. Migraine Intervention with STARFlex® Technology. EuroPCRonline website.

31. Wilmshurst P, Dowson A, Muir K, Mullen M, Nightingale S. The prevalence and size of persistent foramen ovale in migraine patients: preliminary results from the Migraine Intervention with STARFlex® Technology (MIST) Trial. Circulation 2005; 112(suppl 2):II–648(abstract).

32. Steele JG, Nath PU, Burn J, Porteous MEM. An association between migrainous aura and hereditary hemorrhagic telangiectasia. Headache 1993; 33:145–8.
33. Silvestrini M, Cupini LM, Calabresi P, Floris R, Bernardi G. Migraine with aura-like syndrome due to arteriovenous malformations. The clinical value of transcranial Doppler in early diagnosis. Cephalalgia 1992; 12:115–19.
34. Wilmshurst PT, Nightingale S, Walsh KP, Morrison WL. Effect on migraine of closure of cardiac right-to-left shunts to prevent recurrence of decompression illness or stroke or for hemodynamic reasons. Lancet 2000; 356:1648–51.
35. Morandi E, Anzola GP, Angeli S, Melzi G, Onorato E. Transcatheter closure of patent foramen ovale: A new migraine treatment. J Interven Cardiol 2003; 16:39–42.
36. Schwerzmann M, Wiher S, Nedeltchev K et al. Percutaneous closure of patent foramen ovale reduces the frequency of migraine attacks. Neurology 2004; 62:1399–1401.
37. Post MC, Thijs V, Herroelen L, Budts WIHL. Closure of a patent foramen ovale is associated with a decrease in prevalence of migraine. Neurology 2004; 62:1439–40.
38. Reisman M, Jesurum JT, Spencer MP et al. Migraine relief following transcatheter closure of patent foramen ovale. J Am Coll Cardiol 2004; 43(supplement A):376A (abstract).
39. Azarbal B, Tobis J, Suh W, Chan V, Dao C, Gaster R. Association of interatrial shunts and migraine headaches. Impact of transcatheter closure. J Am Coll Cardiol 2005; 45:489–92.
40. Reisman M, Christofferson RD, Jesurum J et al. Migraine headache relief after transcatheter closure of patent foramen ovale. J Am Coll Cardiol 2005; 45:493–5.
41. Gaddum JH, Hebb CO, Silver A, Swan AAB. 5-Hydroxytryptamine. Pharmacologic action and destruction in perfused lungs. Q J Exp Physiol 1953; 38:255–62.
42. Bateman DN. Triptans and migraine. Lancet 2000; 355:860–1.
43. Peto R, Gray R, Collins R et al. Randomized trial of prophylactic daily aspirin in British male doctors. BMJ 1988; 296:313–16.
44. Gamberini G, D'Alessandro R, Labriola E et al. Further evidence on the association of mitral valve prolapse and migraine. Headache 1984; 24:39–40.
45. Kern RZ, Asa S. Left atrial myxoma presenting as migraine with aura: a VIP-induced syndrome? Headache 2005; 45:251–4.
46. Wilmshurst PT, Nightingale S, Walsh KP, Morrison WL. Clopidogrel reduces migraine with aura after transcatheter closure of persistent foramen ovale and atrial septal defects. Heart 2005; 91:1173–5.
47. Sharifi M, Dehghani M, Mehdipour M, Al-Bustami O, Emrani F, Burks J. Intense migraine secondary to percutaneous closure of atrial septal defects. J Interven Cardiol 2005; 18:181–3.

5

Echocardiography of atrial septal defects

George R Sutherland and Robert H Anderson

Introduction   •   Four types of defect   •   Choice of imaging   •   The flap valve of the oval fossa

INTRODUCTION

The morphology of the atria and the interatrial septum is complex.[1,2] Echocardiography is the front-line approach to determining the integrity of the atrial septum. The combined use of high-resolution 2-D imaging, color Doppler and pervenous contrast echocardiography using either the precordial or trans-esophageal approach will usually define whether the atrial septum is intact or not, and if not, will characterize the morphology(s) of any defects. If doubt exists about the precise nature of a defect or if the morphology of pulmonary or systemic venous drainage needs to be clarified then a cardiac magnetic resonance imaging study should be undertaken. Angiography is usually superfluous but may be of value in detecting arterio-venous fistulae which may allow the early appearance of pervenous contrast in the left atrium and thus give the false impression of a right to left atrial shunt in patients with an intact atrial septum.

FOUR TYPES OF DEFECT

Defects in the atrial septum are classically subdivided into four distinct morphologic types: i) partial atrioventricular septal defects (ostium primum defects), ii) defects which involve the margins of the oval fossa – the so-called secundum atrial septal defect, iii) defects of the atrial roof – the sinus venosus defects and iv) defects which border the opening of the coronary sinus, the rare coronary sinus defects. In addition, the flap valve of the oval fossa may itself be partially deficient, fenestrated or aneurysmal with multiple fenestrations. It may also be probe patent[3] (Figures 5.1–5.3) and thus allowing flow to cross it if either atrial pressure is abnormally raised or if dilatation of either (or both) atria occurs. All of the above interatrial communications have the ability to allow bi-directional shunting of blood across them and thus are potential conduits of paradoxical emboli. However, only secundum defects and defects involving the flap valve of the oval fossa are suitable for device closure. Thus, the first role of echocardiography is to define defect morphology if shunting at atria is suspected.

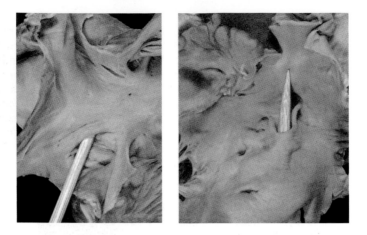

Figure 5.1   A morphologic specimen illustrating probe patency of the flap valve of the oval fossa and its complex morphology. Left panel: The oval fossa visualized from the right side with the probe entering a patent flap valve. Right panel: The probe seen to exit on the left atrial side through a tunnel-like probe patent flap valve.

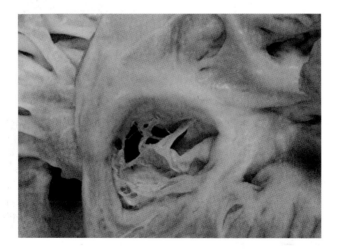

Figure 5.2   Multiple fenestrations of an aneurysmal flap valve of the oval fossa.

Partial atrioventricular septal defects are characterized by an absence of the membranous portion of the atrioventricular septum.[4] This in turn is frequently associated with incomplete formation and separation of the common atrioventricular valve into distinct mitral and tricuspid valves which are offset one from the other in the normal heart with the mitral valve septal leaflet inserted into the central fibrous body at the base of the interatrial septum. The insertion of the septal tricuspid valve into the central fibrous body is lower and separated from the mitral insertion by the atrioventricular septum. In normal hearts this offsetting of septal leaflet insertion is an obvious feature, best seen by cardiac ultrasound using an apical transducer position and scanning through the four-chamber view from back to front (Figure 5.4). This offsetting is frequently absent in partial atrioventricular septal defects, in which a common anterior and posterior atrioventricular leaflet straddles the crest of the interventricular septum at the same level (Figure 5.4). Immediately above the common bridging leaflets lies the ostium primum defect in the atrial septum. This may be of variable size (Figure 5.5). The defect may be large and extend to the area of the oval fossa with the flap valve being virtually absent. In other hearts the defect may be small and

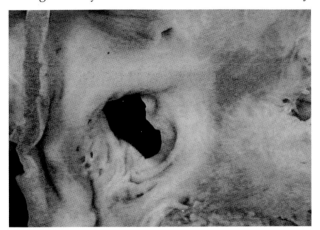

Figure 5.3 A secundum septal defect with deficiency of the central and superior parts of the flap valve of the oval fossa.

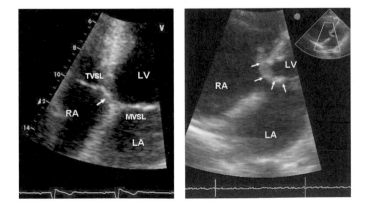

Figure 5.4 Left panel: The normal structure of the atrioventricular junction visualized in a precordial four-chamber view. The mitral valve septal leaflet (MVSL) is seen to be inserted at the base of the atrial septum. The atrioventricular membranous septum (large arrow) is seen to separate the MVSL from the tricuspid valve septal leaflet (TVSL). The TVSL is inserted more apically into the central fibrous body. Right panel: The abnormal structure of the atrioventricular junction found in a primum atrial septal defect. The atrioventricular membranous septum is absent and the common anterior leaflet is seen to form the lower border of the primum defect in the atrial septum.

associated with patency of the foramen ovale or one or more secundum atrial septal defects. In virtually all hearts with ostium primum atrial septal defects, the malformation of the left component of the common valve results in a defect in the leaflets which allows blood to pass from the left ventricle in systole into the left atrium and/or across the primum atrial septal defect into the right atrium. If the right component of the common valve is similarly deficient and pulmonary artery/right ventricular–left atrial shunt through the primum atrial septal defect. Interatrial shunting will also be present – typically this is predominantly left to right atrial but virtually all primum defects have a small right-to-left shunt during the cardiac cycle.

Transthoracic echocardiography will virtually always define the morphology of a partial atrioventricular septal defect and determine the patterns of intracardiac shunting. Associated anomalies are also usually well defined without recourse to transesophageal imaging. As this spectrum of defects is not suitable for device closure it is unnecessary to dwell further on their morphology here.

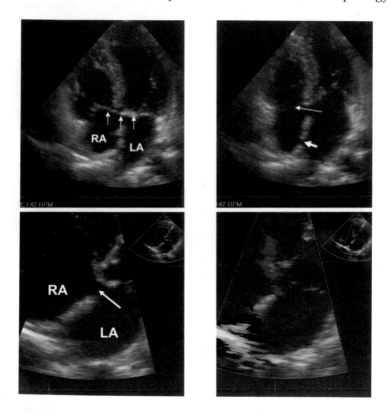

Figure 5.5   The typical ultrasound features of an ostium primum atrial septal defect. Upper left panel: The common bridging anterior leaflet (arrowed). Upper right panel: There are two defects in the interatrial septum. The defect immediately above the atrioventricular junction is the ostium primum defect (thinner arrow). There is a second defect in the secundum position (thicker arrow). Lower left panel: An expanded view of the ostium primum atrial septal defect. Lower right panel: Color flow Doppler image of the interatrial shunt through the primum defect. RA = right atrium, LA = left atrium.

Sinus venosus atrial septal defects are the third most common atrial septal defect but are not true atrial septal defects but rather are defects of the atrial wall. By far the most common form is the superior defect which is a defect of the atrial roof, and is typically sited at the junction of the superior caval vein with the heart. There is also an associated constant anomaly of pulmonary venous drainage with the right upper pulmonary vein draining directly to the superior caval vein just above the superior rim of the defect. Other anomalies of drainage of the right-sided pulmonary veins may occur in association with this type of defect, but are rare. The left-sided pulmonary veins are almost invariably normal in their drainage pattern.

The inferior form of a sinus venosus defect is very rare. The defect is sited at the orifice of the inferior caval vein. This defect is also associated with anomalies of drainage of the right-sided pulmonary veins which may drain either to the inferior vena cava or to the hepatic vein.

Sinus venosus defects are rarely visualized directly from a transthoracic transducer position (Figure 5.6). Using this imaging approach, all the features of

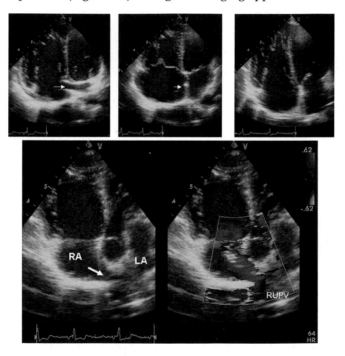

Figure 5.6   A sinus venosus defect. The upper three panels suggest that the interatrial septum is intact, but an intracardiac shunt is present because of the very dilated right ventricle. In the upper left panel the coronary sinus is seen draining normally to the right atrium (arrowed). In the middle upper panel a secundum atrial septum appears intact (arrowed). This is also the case when scanning more anteriorly (upper right panel). However, when scanning posteriorly a defect was seen in the upper atrial wall (large arrow). Color flow Doppler confirmed flow across the defect from a superior vena cava which overrode the defect and to which the right upper pulmonary vein (RUPV) drained. It is unusual to identify a sinus venosus defect from the precordial transducer position. A transesephageal study (see Figure 5.7) is normally required to characterize sinus venosus defects.

a significant atrial left-to-right shunt will be present: volume overload of the right ventricle, a dilated main pulmonary artery with increased flow and a moderate elevation of pulmonary pressure. Yet from the praecordial approach the inter-atrial septum will appear intact and pulmonary venous drainage may appear normal. This paradox should alert the investigator to the possible presence of a sinus venosus defect. The atrial septum should then be visualized from the subcostal position. Only from here will both the superior and inferior defects be visualized and characterized. The superior defect will be seen at the superior caval vein–right atrial junction with apparent 'over-ride' of the superior caval vein over the interatrial septum. This is best visualized using the subcostal four-chamber view. By then rotating the transducer gradually clockwise, the site of abnormal drainage of the superior right pulmonary vein to the superior caval vein will be detected. The use of color Doppler will facilitate this investigation and should routinely be used.

In children and adults the subcostal window may not allow adequate visualization of the superior form of sinus venosus defect. In such cases, a transesophageal study may be appropriate (Figure 5.7). These defects are well characterized by cardiac magnetic resonance imaging.

The rare inferior form of the defect is also well characterized by sub-costal imaging, but the associated anomalies of pulmonary venous drainage may be more difficult to define. A cardiac magnetic resonance study should be performed in all such cases where echocardiography fails to clearly define the morphology of the drainage of the right pulmonary veins.

Coronary sinus atrial septal defects are very rare anomalies. Few reports exist on the use of echocardiography to define their morphology. The interatrial defect

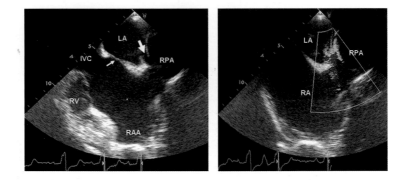

Figure 5.7   The characteristic transesophageal findings of a sinus venosus defect. Such defects are best visualized in an ultrasound plane which visualizes the right atrium and the superior and inferior vena cavae in their long axis. The superior sinus venosus defect in the atrial wall (large arrow) will be visualized lying immediately below the right pulmonary artery. It will be clearly seen to be separated from the oval fossa (small arrow) by the atrial wall with its interposed layer of fatty tissue. Flow across the defect is readily confirmed by the use of color flow mapping (right panel). When such defects are visualized a search should be made for the drainage of the right upper pulmonary vein. This is typically to the superior vena cava at its junction with the right atrium and is best visualized during a transesophageal study by the use of scanning through a series of short-axis planes at the junction of the superior vena cava with the atria. RPA = right pulmonary artery, RAA = right atrial appendage, IVC = inferior vena cava.

is sited around the mouth of an unroofed coronary sinus which also receives blood from a persistent left superior caval vein. The defect itself is difficult to visualize from the transthoracic approach and normally is better seen from a subcostal transducer position. The clue to the ultrasound diagnosis of these defects is the visualization of a very dilated coronary sinus which receives a persistent left superior caval vein. In combination with these two anomalies, the right heart will show all the features of volume overload, typical of an atrial septal defect. To distinguish simple drainage of a persistent left superior caval vein to a normally roofed coronary sinus from a coronary sinus atrial septal defect, a per venous contrast injection should be given into a left arm vein. Where a coronary sinus atrial septal defect is present bubbles from the left caval vein will be seen to enter the left atrium from the unroofed coronary sinus, before the right atrium is opacified. This unique pattern is unique to a coronary sinus atrial septal defect.

Secundum atrial septal defects are defects which involve (and are restricted to) the margins of the oval fossa and its flap valve (Figure 5.8). They may be highly variable in their morphology[5,6] and may extend to involve the superior, anterior, posterior and inferior rims of the oval fossa. They may be single or multiple. The flap valve of the oval fossa may be partially or wholly deficient or may be fenestrated or aneurysmal (with or without fenestrations) (Figure 5.9). Secundum defects may co-exist with all other forms of atrial septal defects.

In terms of device closure, it is essential that an imaging technique not only both ascertains the presence and morphology of a secundum defect, but also defines its spatial relationship to contiguous structures and excludes associated abnormalities within the atria or abnormalities of pulmonary venous drainage.[7] Both echocardiography and cardiac magnetic resonance imaging are suited for this, but each has it relative strengths and weaknesses.

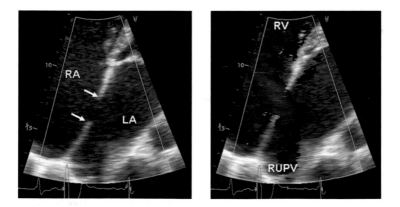

Figure 5.8 The typical findings in a moderate-sized secundum atrial septal defect. The flap valve of the oval fossa is deficient and a 2.2 cm defect is visualized. The presence of the defect is confirmed by color flow mapping. RA = right atrium, LA = left atrium, RUPV = right upper pulmonary vein.

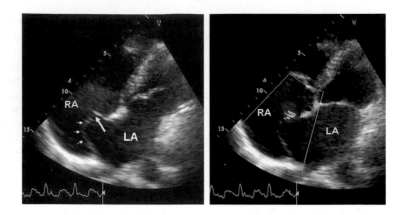

Figure 5.9 An aneurysm of the interatrial septum (small arrows) with a large fenestration. Left-to-right shunting across the aneurysm is seen on color flow Doppler (left-hand panel).

CHOICE OF IMAGING

Echocardiography is usually the first imaging approach which is used. Secundum atrial defects may be suspected following a routine clinical examination and/or chest X-ray, but may be an incidental finding during a routine echocardiographic examination. From either a transthoracic or subcostal transducer position an area of ultrasound 'drop-out' representing a defect will be seen involving the borders of the oval fossa. A continuous scan through either a transthoracic or subcostal four-chamber view will normally define both the size and morphology of the defect(s) and its relationship to the coronary sinus, aortic root and superior caval vein orifice. Such a scan should attempt also to define the relationship of the defect to the venous valves within the right atrium, as even the most experienced echocardiographer can mistake these structures as part of the rim of a secundum atrial septal defect and thus mis-size a defect. Scanning through the four-chamber plane should, in patients with good image quality, identify if more than one secundum defect is present. A series of transthoracic, subcostal, and supra-sternal imaging planes should be used to define the morphology of pulmonary venous drainage.

Where image quality is poor, or in patients in whom a false-positive area of 'drop-out' in the atrial septum is suspected, the addition of Doppler color flow imaging may be helpful. In hearts in which a broad band of color flow is seen to cross the atrial septum within or around the oval fossa, then a secundum defect may be inferred (or confirmed). Equally well in hearts with evidence of right heart volume overload and an apparently intact secundum septum the presence of color flow across the atrial septum may provide convincing evidence that a defect is present. This is especially true if flow is seen to cross the secundum septum from a subcostal imaging position. However, ultrasound artefacts may give rise to the spurious appearance of color flow across the secund septum. This is especially true when imaging from a transthoracic position, when the ultrasound beam is aligned parallel to the atrial septum and color flow data may be incorrectly displayed within an intact atrial septum. However, in older children or adults, the situation frequently exists that a small defect in the atrial septum can neither be visualized with certainty nor excluded. In such cases a pervenous echo contrast study may be the next recourse (Figure 5.10). The technique used for such a study will be described later in the section on determining the integrity of the flap valve of the oval fossa. If the presence or absence of a defect of the secundum cannot be ascertained by a routine ultra-sound examination or a contrast study suggests a significant defect is present, but its precise size and/or morphology is not well defined, then either a trans-esophageal echo or a cardiac magnetic resonance study may be performed.

Transesophageal echocardiography is an unpleasant procedure for the patient, but is especially so in adolescents and young adults, even when performed with adequate sedation. It is usually well tolerated in adults over 35 years of age with adequate sedation. In children and adolescents such studies normally require general anesthesia or heavy sedation. The above may dictate the investigators choice of whether to use transesophageal echo or to proceed to magnetic resonance imaging to define defect morphology.

The atrial septum is well seen by multiplane transesophageal imaging. With its high spatial resolution in normal hearts, it can define the unfolding of the atrial walls and their intervening fat pad at the superior rim of the oval fossa. It can also better define the site of drainage of the pulmonary veins, the site of drainage of the coronary sinus and the relationship of the flap valve of the oval fossa to the venous valves of the right atrium compared to precordial echocar-diography. Any defect of the flap valve of the oval fossa will normally be easily

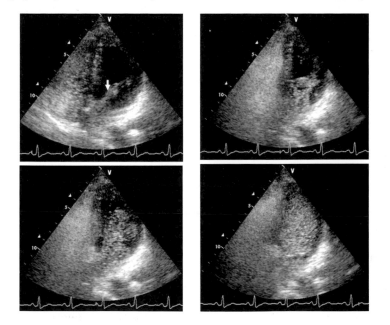

Figure 5.10 A pervenous contrast study to determine possible patency of an apparently intact atrial septum on transthoracic imaging. Following a Valsalva maneuver (upper left panel) contrast is seen to enter the left atrium from the right atrium (arrowed). The further three frames show the significant right-to-left shunt produced immediately following the Valsalva maneuver.

visualized as will a defect of the rim of the fossa. Scanning the defect through a number of planes will determine its extension and relationship with contiguous structures and maximal defect dimensions (antero-posterior and infero-superior) can be measured with accuracy. Defects which involve the superior-anterior rim are the most common with defects extending posteriorly being the least common.[6] When defects are deemed size-wise to be suitable for device closure, then a careful study of the defect rims should be made to make certain there is sufficient rim tissue to allow stable device placement and that contiguous structures such as the coronary sinus, tricuspid valve and right upper pulmonary vein will be unobstructed by device placement. The pressure of a second, or multiple defects, must also be excluded. It is all too easy for the novice investigator to be pleased that he has visualized one defect and to forget to search for others. Where one (or more) defects are visualized by gray-scale imaging and flow across the defect(s) confirmed by color Doppler, then a contrast echo study is of little added value. Similarly, if the defect is fully characterized by a transesophageal study and is defined to be too big for device closure but is suitable for surgery, then there is little benefit in a correlative magnetic resonance imaging study. However, if ambiguities exist or the transesophageal study is technically suboptimal, then a magnetic resonance imaging study should be performed.

Three-dimensional imaging of secundum defect morphology should be the optimal approach to defining these defects suitable for device closure. This can be attempted using either ultrasound[8] or magnetic resonance imaging. However, both approaches have their limitations. This is especially true of current ultrasound technologies. The first 3-D ultrasound attempts to define atrial septal defect morphology were based on single-plane transesophageal transducers in which a stepping motor was used to control the rotation of the ultrasound array. The theoretical advantage of this approach was the relatively high spatial resolution of the image, but this advantage was lost as most of the ultrasound data (as high as 95%) had to be discarded in the reconstruction of the surface-rendered images. This approach has now been largely abandoned. With the development of real-time 3-D matrix probes, transthoracic 3-D reconstruction of defect morphology is theoretically possible. However, current real-time 3-D technology has inherently poor spatial resolution and is fraught with image artefacts. It remains less than optimal in defining 3-D defect morphology compared to 3-D magnetic resonance imaging.

THE FLAP VALVE OF THE OVAL FOSSA

In the normal heart, the thin flap of the oval fossa closes any potential interatrial communication. However, in utero this flap valve is widely patent allowing the obligatory right-to-left atrial shunting of blood necessary for survival of the fetus. Following birth, and flow through the lungs, the pressure within the left atrium will become greater than that in the right and the flap valve will be closed. The time at which this happens will vary and will depend on the normal fall in right atrial pressure. However, by three months of age, no left-to-right shunting should occur in the normal infant's heart. Yet the flap valve may remain potentially patent in most hearts into late childhood or adolescence.

This can be confirmed by the ease with which it is possible to cross a probe patent foramen ovale at catheterization in most young children. In adults, potential patency of a normal flap valve is not uncommon – the exact incidence is unclear and will be determined by the provocation used to attempt to open the flap valve, the sensitivity of the imaging technique used and the presence of raised atrial pressure and atrial dilatation.

In addition, the flap valve itself may not be a simple structure, but may be three dimensional, being tunnel-like in over one third of cases. It may also have continuity with the venous valves within the right atrium. Within the left atrium the flap valve's inferior rim will frequently be seen in transesophageal echocardiography to extend down to just above the septal aspect of the left atrioventricular junction.

The flap valve may also be aneurysmal and highly mobile. Such aneurysmal flap valves may be intact or have multiple fenestrations within them. It may be very difficult to exclude such multiple small defects even on transesophageal imaging if atrial pressures are equal and flow is non-turbulent across them. In such situations only pervenous contrast echocardiography may confirm the presence of uni- or bi-directional atrial shunting.

Aneurysms of the flap valve of the atrial septum if large and mobile have been associated with a higher than expected incidence of systemic embolic events. This may simply be due to right-to-left shunting across the septum due to the increased incidence of defects within the flap valve itself, or to the presence of a small associated secundum atrial septal defect, but case reports have clearly identified a possible thrombogenic propensity within large mobile aneurysms of the flap valve which have been shown to contain thrombus.

Large aneurysms of the atrial septum are frequently visualized using standard precordial echocardiography. They may be mobile, moving to point to within either the left or right atrium, during the respiratory cycle. They may also be fixed with the direction in which they point being determined by either a constant direction of flow across them or by a constant difference in atrial pressures. If precordial or subcostal image quality is poor then they can be detected by a transesophageal study.

With the increasing awareness of the potential role of patency of the flap valve of the oval fossa in patients with unexplained systemic embolic events more and more patients with neurological events or unexplained symptoms are being referred to cardiologists for investigations of the integrity of the atrial septum. A pervenous contrast echocardiographic study is now routine in all such cases (Figure 5.10). This should be performed in conjunction with a Valsalva maneuver which is used to rapidly elevate right atrial pressure and thus test the patency of the flap valve. A solution of agitated saline or a mixture of agitated blood and saline will act as a cheap and effective contrast agent. There is no need to resort to the current range of expensive pharmaceutical contrast agents – they offer no diagnostic benefits. Likewise it is unnecessary to proceed immediately to a transesophageal study in such cases. In the authors experience a Valsalva maneuver is much better performed in an unsedated patient and may not be performed satisfactorily during a transesophageal study. Thus, the first approach to defining potential patency of the oval fossa should be a pervenous contrast echo. Only if bubbles cross the atrial septum during a properly performed Valsalva maneuver should a transesophageal study be undertaken to determine the morphology and site(s) of any defect. Such an appropriate clinical approach will obviate the need for the countless unnecessary transesophageal studies that are currently being carried out to determine whether the foramen ovale is patent.

REFERENCES

1. Anderson RH, Webb S, Brown NA. Clinical anatomy of the atrial septum with reference to its developmental components. Clin Anat 1999; 12:362–74.
2. Ho SY, Anderson RH, Sanchez-Quintana D. Gross structure of the atriums: more than an anatomic curiosity? Pacing Clin Electrophysiol 2002; 25(3):342–50.
3. Hagen PT, Scholz DG, Edwards WD. Incidence and size of patent foramen ovale during the first 10 decades of life: an autopsy study of 965 normal hearts. Mayo Clin Proc 1984; 59(1):17–20.
4. Flacao S, Daliento L, Ho SY, Rigby ML, Anderson RH. Cross sectional echocardiographic assessment of the extent of the atrial septum relative to the atrioventricular junction in atrioventricular septal defect. Heart 1999; 81:199–205.
5. Chan KC, Godman MJ. Morphological variations of fossa ovalis atrial septal defects (Secundum): feasibility for transcutaneous closure with the clam-shell device. Br Heart J 1993; 69:52–5.
6. Prokselj K, Kozelj M, Zadnik V, Podnar T. Echocardiographic characteristics of secundum-type atrial septal defects in adult patients; implications for percutaneous closure using amplatzer septal occluders. J Am Soc Echocardiogr 2004; 17(11):1167–72.
7. Said HG, McMahon CJ, Mullins CE et al. Patent foramen ovale morphology and impact on percutaneous device closure. Paediatr Cardiol 2005; 26(1):62–5.
8. Franke A, Kuhl HP, Rulands D et al. Quantitative analysis of the morphology of secundum-type atrial septal defects and their dynamic change using transoesophageal three-dimensional echocardiography. Circulation 1997; 4(96) (9 Suppl):323–7.

6

Intracardiac echocardiography of the interatrial septum

Michael J Mullen

Introduction • **Devices and procedures** • **Guiding closure** • **Summary**

INTRODUCTION

Echocardiography is an important element in the assessment of patients with defects of the intra-atrial septum and in guiding device closure. To date this has normally been performed using a combination of transthoracic and transesophageal echocardiography. These techniques are limited by poor resolution and inadequate quality of imaging in the case of TTE and the invasive nature of TEE, which usually necessitates the use of general anesthesia or deep sedation. The development and evolution of intracardiac echocardiography offers a new technique that allows high-quality invasive imaging of the interatrial septum in non-sedated patients, now that transcatheter closure of atrial septal defects has been established as a safe and effective treatment with good results.[1-3]

The initial assessment of patients for device closure of defects of the interatrial septum usually involves a combination of physical examination and transthoracic echocardiography. Dilation of the right heart is the hallmark of atrial septal defects. Using modern echocardiographic systems with harmonic imaging, skilled operators can almost always determine the nature and size of the defect. Ostium primum and sinus venosus defects are more complex defects not suitable for device closure and these can normally be readily excluded by transthoracic echocardiography. The size and position of secundum defects helps determine the suitability for device closure.

The recent development of minaturized catheter-mounted transducers that allow direct echocardiographic imaging from within the heart itself – intracardiac echocardiography – has added greatly to the tools available to guide percutaneous device closure.[4] The catheters are advanced from a peripheral vein (normally femoral) and the majority of imaging performed from the right atrium where excellent views of the interatrial septum are acquired. Such catheters can be used to guide transseptal puncture[5] and have been shown to be a useful alternative to general anesthesia and transesophageal echocardiography in guiding percutaneous device closure of the atrial septum.[6,7]

DEVICES AND PROCEDURE

To date, two separate systems have been available. The Boston-Scientific Ultra ICE system has a 9 MHz transducer mounted on a 9Fr catheter. The transducer is advanced to the RA utilizing a long sheath technique. Rotation of the transducer through 360 degrees allows a two-dimensional transverse image of the heart to be acquired. Withdrawal of and advancing the transducer in a cranio-caudal fashion allows high-resolution imaging of the interatrial septum. The system is limited in that it only offers two-dimensional imaging and is non-steerable.

In contrast, the Siemens Acunav system (Figure 6.1) has a 64-element phased array transducer positioned on the tip of a 10Fr steerable catheter. This system provides a sector image similar to those seen with TTE and TEE. The transducer has full color flow and Doppler facilities and operates between 5.5 MHz and 10 MHz allowing adjustment of the image for high resolution or penetration and color flow mapping at lower frequencies. The catheter tip can be steered through the heart using a combination of rotation and quadridirectional steering mounted on the manifold. The recent development of an 8Fr system and approval for use in the left heart has further expanded the utility of this technology in children.

The ICE catheter is usually introduced via the right femoral vein using a separate 11Fr or 8Fr sheath depending on the system being used. Occasionally the catheter may be introduced from the jugular or subclavian veins. The catheter is guided to the right atrium by direct fluoroscopy or using the ultrasound image. From within the right atrium the entire heart may be imaged. Once the catheter tip is positioned within the right atrium it is usually easy to identify the tricuspid valve by rotating the catheter approximately 30 degrees clockwise from the anterior position. This is often referred to as the home view as it is easy to achieve without manipulation of the catheter and from this position the catheter can be steered to image the rest of the heart. From the home view the catheter is further rotated clockwise to image the right ventricular outflow tract and aorta in long axis. Behind the aorta the interatrial septum is imaged for the first time. The inferior vena cava tends to direct the catheter directly towards the oval fossa and, therefore, the catheter tip usually needs to be gently flexed posteriorly, using the controls on the manifold, to fully image the interatrial septum. From

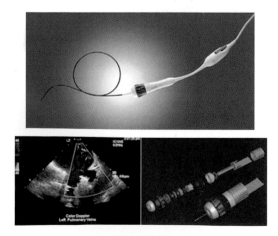

Figure 6.1 The Siemens Acuson AcuNav Intracardiac Echo Catheter.

this position the inferior and superior limits of the septum may be assessed by advancing and withdrawing the catheter between the superior and inferior vena cava. These areas, which may be difficult to image with TEE, are particularly well seen using ICE. The left pulmonary veins can be imaged on the far wall of the left atrium, whilst the right pulmonary veins are identified by further clockwise rotation of the catheter as they enter the left atrium behind the origin of the superior vena cava. The right pulmonary artery courses superiorly to the right pulmonary veins. Each structure may be individually assessed using two-dimensional imaging, color flow, pulse wave, and continuous wave Doppler (Figure 6.2). A short axis view of the interatrial septum can be obtained by further posterior flexion of the catheter and rotation towards the tricuspid valve, and by using the left and right controls the image may be further optimized.

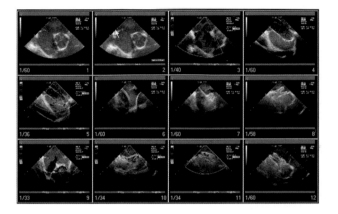

Figure 6.2 Top panel from left to right: Short axis view with the aortic valve in the center, showing a secundum atrial septal defect, the same with markers for measurement, the same with color Doppler, a long axis view showing an Amplatzer® sizing balloon occluding flow. Middle panel from left to right: Long axis view showing sizing balloon with minimal shunt across the defect – measuring the 'stop-flow' diameter, Long axis view showing an Amplatzer® delivery cable across an atrial septal defect, the left atrial disk of an Amplatzer® septal occluder being deployed, both disks of an Amplatzer® septal occluder deployed. Bottom panel from left to right: color Doppler flow across an atrial septal defect, a fully deployed and correctly positioned Amplatzer® septal occluder with color flow seen in the device (normal just after deployment) and some flow around the edge superiorly – due to tension on the loading cable, fully deployed and released Amplatzer® septal occluder with and without color flow Doppler.

GUIDING CLOSURE

Using these simple maneuvers the whole of the interatrial septum may be adequately assessed. The type, size, and number of defects may be determined and device deployment monitored. Deployment of atrial septal closure devices is often best imaged using the short axis imaging plane. This particularly facilitates imaging of device deployment at the aortic rim which is often deficient in patients with an ASD. The utility of ICE in guiding closure of ASD has been determined in a number of studies. ICE has been shown to be accurate in the assessment of ASD and guiding their closure reliably, detecting device malposition, additional defects, and other procedural complications (Figures 6.3–6.5). We found no limitation in the use of ICE during closure of large or multiple defects, and ICE may be more effective than other imaging modalities in assessing inferiorly positioned defects. Recently reported benefits include reduced procedural and fluoroscopy times, with ICE-guided closure of ASD benefiting both patients and the efficient use of catheter laboratory resources. The avoidance of general anesthesia facilitates rapid patient recovery, mobilization, and discharge.

The closure of patent foramen ovale presents different challenges to that of ASD. Defects that are difficult to detect using TEE, particularly if performed under general anesthesia (GA), are often seen by ICE, and the anatomy of the defect may be determined. A contrast echo may be performed when, unlike during TEE, the patient is fully able to perform provocative maneuvers which increases the likelihood of successfully identifying the shunt. We have seen a

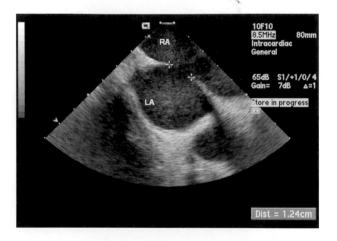

Figure 6.3 Intracardiac echo imaging demonstrating measurement of a secundum atrial septal defect.

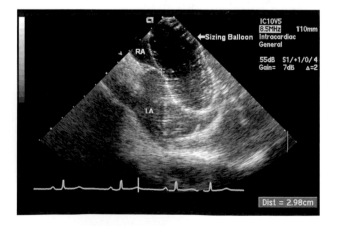

Figure 6.4 Intracardiac echo imaging demonstrating measurement of an Amplatzer® sizing balloon inflated across a secundum atrial septal defect.

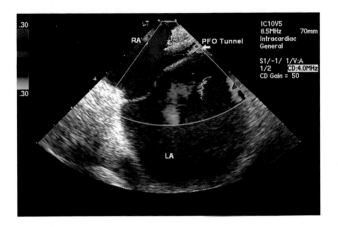

Figure 6.5 Intracardiac echo imaging with color Doppler demonstrating a small shunt through a tunnel-like patent foramen ovale.

number of patients in whom the defect could not be identified with TEE whilst under GA, in whom we have subsequently successfully identified and closed the defect using ICE. If appropriate, ICE may also be used to guide a transseptal puncture, when identification of the site of tenting of the septum facilitates an accurate and safe puncture.

SUMMARY

Modern ICE systems represent a significant advance over TEE in assessing and guiding the closure of defects of the interatrial septum. Intracardiac echocardiography provides high-quality and complete imaging of the defect in the fully conscious patient avoiding the need for general anesthesia or sedation. As the number of procedures increases, ICE will likely become the standard method for guiding these procedures.

REFERENCES

1. Chan KC, Godman MJ, Walsh K et al. Transcatheter closure of atrial septal defect and inter-atrial communications with a new self expanding nitinol double disc device (Amplatzer septal occluder): multicentre UK experience. Heart 1999; 82:300–6.
2. Justo RN, Nyaken DG , Boutin C et al. Clinical impact of transcatheter closure of secundum atrial septal defects with the double umbrella device. Am J Cardiol 1996; 77:889–92.
3. Carminati M, Giusti S, Hausdorf G et al. A European muticentretic experience using the CardioSEAL and STARFlex double umbrella devices to close interatrial communications holes within the oval fossa. Cardiol Young 2000; 10:519–26.
4. Bruce CJ, Packer DL, Seward JB. Intracardiac Doppler hemodynamics and flow: new vector, phased array ultrasound-tipped catheter. Am J Cardiol 1999; 83:1509–12, A9.
5. Daoud EG, Kalbfleish SJ, Hummel JD. Intracardiac echocardiography to guide transeptal left heart catheterization for radiofrequency catheter ablation. J Cardiovasc Electrophysiol 1999; 10:358–63.
6. Hijazi ZM, Wang Z, Cao QL et al. Transcatheter closure of atrial septal defects and patent foramen ovale under intracardiac echocardiographic guidance: feasibility and comparison with transoesophageal echocardiography. Catheter Cardiovasc Interv 2001; 1:52:194–9.
7. Mullen MJ, Dias BF, Walker F, Siu SC, Benson LN, McLaughlin PR. Intracardiac echocardiography guided device closure of atrial septal defects. J Am Coll Cardiol 2003; 41:285–92.

Section 2
Techniques and devices

7

Technique of percutaneous closure of the atrial septal defect and patent foramen ovale

Kevin P Walsh and Anita Dumitrescu

INTRODUCTION

Percutaneous atrial septal defect (ASD) closure is now a routine procedure in many cardiac catheterization laboratories. It has replaced surgery as the method of choice for ASD closure in most patients. The successful percutaneous closure of an ASD requires careful echocardiographic evaluation of the defect, precise device selection, and meticulous implantation technique. Operator experience is a significant factor, as the inexperienced operator will tend to reject potentially suitable patients and oversize devices, which represents a form of false security. It is therefore important that any operator/team have sufficient throughput to develop and maintain skills. It must also be borne in mind, that although trans-catheter closure of the patent foramen ovale (PFO)[1-4] is likely to become an extremely common procedure, the experience gained with PFO closure is unlikely to qualify the operator to close the occasional large atrial septal defect.

PREPARATION

Patients who undergo interventional ASD closure are usually scheduled for a three-day hospital stay. The admission day involves routine blood tests, to rule out coagulation disorders, chest radiograph, ECG (electrocardiogram) and occasionally repeat transthoracic echocardiography (TTE). The interventional cardiac catheterization is performed on the second day, and the patient is discharged on the third day after prior assessment of correct device position and efficacy of defect closure via TTE and chest radiograph.

The use of both transesophageal echocardiography (TEE) and fluoroscopy for ASD-closure ideally requires a still patient. This is best achieved with general anesthesia, particularly in pediatric patients; usually this requires anesthesiology cover. Alternatively, deep sedation with maintained spontaneous breathing can be induced with different types of intravenous anesthetics, such as midazolam, propofol and ketamine, in single or combined administration. Local pharyngeal anesthesia allows for better tolerance of the transesophageal probe in adult patients.

In terms of optimal preparation it is essential that the interventionalist spends sufficient time before starting the procedure with thorough echocardiographic assessment and mapping of the anatomy, rather than paying attention to it only later when running into trouble. This is a crucial aspect of the procedure! A multiplane transesophageal transducer is generally used; however, intracardiac echocardiography (ICE) has found widespread acceptance and use and is easily introduced via femoral venous access. It is available in 8 or 10F (3.2 mm), 5.5 MHz to 10 MHz ultrasound-tipped catheters.[5] Depending on the operator's experience and the defect-morphology, some ASDs are amenable to closure with echocardiographic guidance solely.[6]

Care has to be taken that the patient's body temperature is maintained throughout the procedure. The transesophageal probe is introduced after induction of anesthesia and positioning of the patient. Up to a body weight of 20 kg we use a pediatric probe, above 20 kg, the adult probe. Single plane fluoroscopy is sufficient.

CRITERIA FOR DEVICE CLOSURE

It must be remembered that device occlusion of the defect results in a lifelong implant[7] and although medium and long-term follow-up data are very encouraging, to date there are no very long-term (>10 years) follow-up data available. Appropriate indications for device closure are:

- >7 mm defect persisting beyond infancy
- Qp/Qs > 1.5:1 and/or
- Right ventricular volume overload

Defects suitable for device occlusion are:

- Single or multiple interatrial septal defects
- Multiperforated interatrial septums
- Aneurysms of the interatrial septum with defect
- Patent foramen ovale
- Fenestrated Fontan conduits (after favorable hemodynamic assessment with balloon occlusion).

PERCUTANEOUS VASCULAR ACCESS

Vascular access for ASD closure is obtained percutaneously and catheter insertion performed using Seldinger technique via the right femoral vein and artery, after bilateral surgical disinfection. The left inguinal vessels serve as back-up access, in case of failure to obtain right-sided vascular access or for additional access. Alternative venous access can be achieved via hepatic veins, which requires a special needle and technique. Subclavian and internal jugular veins do not allow for ideal positioning of the delivery sheath and will not be discussed here.

Depending on the patient's age and body weight, in pediatric patients a 6 or 7 French (F) introducer sheath can be used initially for hemodynamic assessment and later exchanged for the recommended delivery sheath-size.

Arterial access may also be obtained for hemodynamic surveillance using, e.g. a 22 or 20F 'Leader catheter'.[8] This arterial line should be securely sewn in.

Once vascular access has been obtained, the patient is given heparin (pediatric patients usually 100 units/kg i.v., adults 5,000 units) as well as the first dose of antibiotic, usually cefuroxime, 30 mg/kg i.v.

TYPES OF ASD-OCCLUDER DEVICES AND DELIVERY SYSTEMS

It is necessary to be familiar with the different devices available and their respective properties in order to choose the adequate introduction and delivery systems for optimal results. The most commonly used devices are:

- Amplatzer® Septal Occluder
- HELEX Septal Occluder
- CardioSEAL® (second and third generation) and its modification, the STARFlex®.

As the Amplatzer® Septal Occluder (ASO) is the only device able to reproduce close, large, hemodynamically significant atrial septal defects, our description of the technique of percutaneous ASD closure will discuss it exclusively.

THE AMPLATZER® SEPTAL OCCLUDER

The conceptual simplicity, easy mechanics and manipulation, the small delivery system and the possibility of repositioning and retrieval in case of incorrect placement any time prior to definitive release, have made the Amplatzer® Septal Occluder, ASO, (AGA, Medical Corp., Golden Valley, MN) the most popular and widely used occlusion device, particularly in pediatric patients, owing to the small delivery system. The device is self-expanding, made of a Nitinol wire-mesh (nickel 55%, titanium 45%), 0.004–0.0075 inches thick, which forms two disks connected by a 3–4 mm thick waist, corresponding to the thickness of the atrial septum.[9] Slight inclination of the two disks towards each other (concave rightward aspect of the left atrial disk) improves the 'grasp' onto the septal rim(s). Three Dacron polyester patches, sewn inside the disks and waist with a polyester thread, instigate thrombus formation following the principle of Virchow's triad, with laminar blood flow being disturbed and slowed and surface roughened, characterizing the 'sealing' properties of the device.

Nitinol is superelastic yet lacks plastic properties, resulting in an exceptional quality called 'shape memory'. This shape memory is responsible for the unchanged reshaping (elastic quality) of the ASO without deformation (plastic quality) after loading it into the delivery system in a compressed, linear configuration.

Table 7.1 Left and right atrial rims for differentatrial septal sizes

Device size (waist diameter)	Left atrial disk	Right atrial disk
4–10 mm	+ 12 mm	+ 8 mm
11–32 mm	+ 14 mm	+ 10 mm
34–40 mm	+ 16 mm	+ 10 mm

Since the atrial septal defects closed with ASO generally have a left-to-right shunt with higher left atrial than right atrial pressures, the disk for the left atrial site is larger than the disk for the right atrial side[5,7] as shown in Table 7.1.

The concept of 'firm septal margins'[7]

The ASO is self-centering but requires sufficient atrial septal rim (5–7 mm) to adjacent structures if it is to be stable and not encroach on valves or veins. Structures to be assessed by transesophageal echocardiography therefore are:

• the atrioventricular valves
• the superior vena cava
• the inferior vena cava
• the right pulmonary veins
• the coronary sinus.

The aortic rim is of lesser importance and can be absent, as the antero-superior atrial wall infolding creates a left atrial recess, where the left atrial disk can be accommodated. This, however, may require a change in the method of implantation, which will be detailed later.

This concept of 'firm margins'[7] is important, as the diameter of the device to be used is often selected on the basis of balloon stretching, and a large device may compress what initially appeared to be adequate margins, resulting in uncomfortable and hazardous proximity to the mitral valve.

How to estimate the size of the device required

Measurement of the left atrial diameter in the subcostal 4-chamber view may allow selection of the maximum diameter device that can be accommodated in a smaller heart. The stretched diameter (using a balloon) plus 14 mm would then have to be within this diameter to permit safe implantation.

The regression line derived from maximum TEE diameter and the balloon stretched diameter is nearly identical to that derived by Rao et al using transthoracic subcostal echocardiographic diameters.[10] Essentially, adding 6 mm to the maximum TEE diameter, in most cases, will give a good estimate of the stretched diameter. This can serve as a useful check during sizing and is helpful when selecting young children for device closure. If the size of device predicted by the maximum TEE or subcostal diameter would be too large to be accommodated in that patient's atrium, the patient can be referred directly for surgery rather than undergoing balloon sizing.[7]

ASO-sizes

The ASO's profile is rather bulky; however, during follow-up studies a reduction in profile has been observed together with excellent endothelialization. It is the only device with an entirely metal surface requiring complete endothelialization. Although there are experimental data showing rapid endothelialization,[9] Nitinol has a long history of clinical use in intravascular implants,[11,12] but there is very little information about the rate of endothelialization of large Nitinol-mesh devices in humans, a fact that theoretically raises questions regarding susceptibility for endocarditis and necessity of long-term endocarditis prophylaxis.

The ASO is available in different sizes determined by the size of its waist.[5] This waist's purpose is to stent the defect, with subsequent thrombotic occlusion of the ASD due to the internal Dacron material.

From 4 to 20 mm waist-size, increments take place in steps of 1 mm, thereafter in 2 mm steps, up to a waist-size size of 40 mm. The size of the delivery system for the Amplatzer® Septal Occluder, depending on the device size used, varies between 6–12 French for devices smaller than 10 mm and for large devices up to 40 mm.[5] Recommendations regarding the size of delivery system are listed in Table 7.2.[5]

Catheterization and determination of defect size

1. A 6 or 7 French end-hole catheter (multipurpose) is flushed, de-aired and introduced to perform a rapid right heart catheterization. Saturations and pressures are sampled from the superior vena cava, pulmonary artery, pulmonary vein, and femoral artery to obtain a Qp/Qs.
2. The catheter is then advanced through the ASD by orientating it posteriorly and to the left. The left atrial septum is profiled using the four-chamber view with 35 degrees cranial/35 degrees left anterior oblique (LAO). An important landmark regarding the entry into the left pulmonary veins is the left main bronchus. The tip of the catheter should point towards the inferior wall of this. Care has to be taken not to manipulate the catheter into the left atrial appendage, which is frail and prone to perforation. (In one elderly lady in our patient collective, a guide-wire perforated the left atrial appendage and entered the pericardial space. This was recognized, the guide-wire withdrawn, repositioned within the pulmonary vein and the procedure continued without complications.[7])

Table 7.2 Recommended size of delivery systems

Delivery system	Atrial septal defect
6F	< 10 mm
7F	10–15 mm
8F	16–20 mm
9F	22–24 mm
10F	26–30 mm
12F	32–40 mm

All catheter manipulations are monitored on fluoroscopy as well as with the chosen echocardiographic method. With TEE the catheter course can some-times be difficult to ascertain since the guide-wire is more echogenic than the catheter. It can be easier to appreciate which defect has been crossed by peeling back the catheter off the wire, while maintaining the wire position. With multiple defects, echocardiographic guidance needs to be particularly thorough to ensure passage through the largest defect.

3. The catheter is now advanced into the medial part of the left upper pulmonary vein, so that a generous length of exchange guide-wire can be left out in the pulmonary vein. If too little guide-wire is placed it will surely fall back into the left atrium or the left atrial appendage.[7]

4. Once a defect has been crossed, it is important to ensure that the wire remains in place until the delivery sheath has been placed, otherwise a large defect may be sized and the large-diameter device delivered into the nearby smaller defect. Occasionally, in patients with multiple large ASDs, it is helpful to inflate a sizing balloon in one defect and then cross the other defect with a catheter introduced from the opposite groin.[7]

Balloon sizing – stop-flow diameter

The original method of balloon sizing was to inflate a latex occlusion or septostomy balloon in the left atrium and gently withdraw it through the atrial septal defect. Under fluoroscopy, the waist forming in the balloon as it pulled through could be measured, or more commonly, the diameter of the balloon was measured in a template (Figure 7.1). This was then taken to be the stretched diameter of the defect. Dynamic balloon sizing is no longer performed and has been replaced by static balloon sizing. Static balloons used currently are the AGA sizing balloon (AGA Medical, Golden Valley, MN) with its calibration markers on the catheter shaft (Figure 7.1) or the NuMed (NuMed, Inc., Hopkinton, NY) PT-OS with internal 1 cm markers for calibration. A 0.035 inch extra-stiff exchange guide-wire is used to exchange the diagnostic catheter for the sizing balloon. The balloon is de-aired and filled with dilute dye (1/3 dye, 2/3 saline solution) or pure saline if echocardiographic guidance is used solely.[6] The sizing balloon is centered within the ASD and inflated, until slight circum-ferential indentation of the balloon is visible, both on fluoroscopy and with echocardiography. The diameter of this waist is measured and taken to be the stretched diameter of the defect. Spot cine measurement needs to be corrected for magnification.[5] The magnification correction can be checked by using the markers within the sizing balloon or on the catheter shaft. To use these markers for correction, the X-ray beam should be positioned orthogonally to them. Unfortunately, this sometimes is at a different angle from the one that profiles the waist. For this reason the ECHO measurement of the waist is usually more reliable. The 45-degree short axis TEE plane shows the waist in the balloon well. It is important to measure the ECHO balloon waist from leading edge to leading edge.

There has been a move away from using the stretched diameter of the defect for selection of the device size, because of the occurrence of erosions of the atrium and aorta (in at least 40 patients or 0.1% of implants) by what was considered to have been oversized implants. It was felt by an expert panel, that

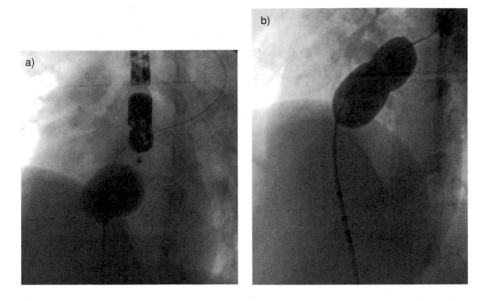

Figure 7.1   Balloon sizing. Figure 7.1a shows the dynamic waist produced on the spherical Meditech sizing balloon as it is gently pulled through the atrial septal defect. Figure 7.1b shows the static indentation on the compliant cigar-shaped balloon inflated in the defect. The radio-opaque markers on the shaft are NOT orthogonal to the X-ray beam. If they are to be used for calibration, the X-ray camera must be rotated (usually 15° LAO) so that the markers become rectangular rather than ellipsoid in shape.

balloon stretching in some of these defects may have resulted in the implantation of an oversized device whose disks rubbed repetitively against the roof of the atrium and adjacent aorta resulting in erosion and tamponade. To avoid this, the stop-flow method for sizing has been advocated. Using color Doppler imaging, the inflation of the balloon is observed until the shunt disappears; the diameter is then measured and considered to be the stop-flow diameter. This diameter is usually smaller than the stretched diameter.

Additional defects are assessed by balloon sizing if they are located far enough from the main defect to require a second device. Often however, an additional small defect will be overlapped by a slightly oversized device in the major defect.

Device selection

Small-diameter defects (< 11 mm) with firm margins can be closed by selecting a device 2–4 mm larger than the defect on two-dimensional (2-D) echo – without recourse to balloon sizing.

For most moderate-sized defects (11–24 mm diameter on 2-D measurement), the device to be implanted is selected on the basis of the stretched diameter of the defect. For most defects, a device with a waist the same size as the stretched diameter of the defect is used. However, for larger defects, 28 to 32 mm stretched diameter, a device with a waist 2 mm larger than the stretched diameter may be chosen to ensure stability. This is because the rim width is fixed at 7 mm in devices with waists ranging from 11 to 32 mm. Thus, with the larger devices the overall device to defect ratio is considerably smaller, so a 32 mm device provides a device to defect ratio of 1.4 compared to a ratio of 2.3 for an 11 mm device.[7]

In large defects in adults (>24 mm on 2-D measurement) balloon sizing is often unrewarding. The AGA 34 mm sizing balloon often cannot be easily stabilized within the defect. We have also had a couple of instances of the balloon tearing the septum and either requiring the implantation of a much larger device or abandonment of the procedure with referral to surgery. We find it much more useful to concentrate on the ECHO assessment of the defect at the beginning of the procedure. The flimsiness of the rims can easily be assessed in multiple planes and the true defect size estimated quite accurately using the width of the color flow jet, which is usually greater than the 2-D diameter of the defect and will give a 'pseudo-stretched' diameter. Multiple measurements with the very flimsy rims excluded, allow a good estimate of the required waist diameter device to seat securely in the defect without being constrained and bulky (Figure 7.2).

Similarly, in small patients (<12 kg) with relatively large defects, balloon sizing is unhelpful and a device can be chosen to match the 2-D diameter of the defect, provided the left atrial disk is not much bigger than the left-sided atrial septal length on the sub-costal four-chamber view.

A major reason for the previous oversizing of devices was the need to use a larger-diameter device to deal with those defects with deficient aortic rims. Because the defect extends antero-superiorly, the device tends to come through the antero-superior part of the defect before the postero-inferior septum is abutted, much like a button coming through a slit-like buttonhole. A larger-diameter device (at least 4 mm larger than the stretched balloon diameter) was required to avoid tilting through the antero-superior portion of the defect. The advent of directional sheaths has markedly simplified the implantation of devices in these defects with deficient aortic rims. The Hausdorf-Lock Sheath

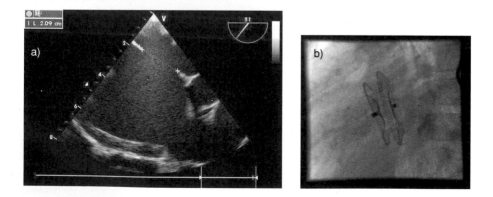

Figure 7.2 Large atrial septal defect with deficient aortic rim. Figure 7.2a shows a transesophageal echo view of a 21 mm defect in a four-year-old boy with a deficient aortic rim. Figure 7.2b shows a lateral fluoroscopic view of an implanted 28 mm Amplatzer® septal occluder. The device was chosen on the basis of the imaging without balloon sizing and implanted using a directional sheath.

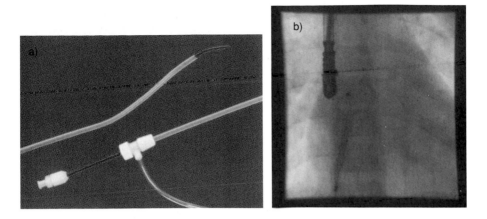

Figure 7.3 Hausdorf Lock Sheath. Figure 7.3a shows the posterior S-shaped curve of the Hausdorf Lock sheath. The side arm should be lying towards the patient's left to orientate the sheath correctly in the left atrium. Figure 7.3b shows an antero-posterior fluoroscopic image of the device being delivered parallel to the atrial septum towards the right upper pulmonary vein.

(Wm Cook Inc.,) has a posterior S-type curve, which orientates the device parallel to the plane of the atrial septum and allows a non-oversized device to be easily implanted in large-diameter defects with deficient aortic rims (Figure 7.3).

Delivery of the device

The appropriate-sized delivery sheath system is flushed, de-aired, and advanced over the wire into the left upper pulmonary vein. It is imperative to avoid air being sucked into the long sheath when the dilator is withdrawn. Due to the low left atrial pressure, air can easily get sucked into the system causing air embolism with transient ST-segment changes and hypotension.[7] Therefore, the dilator is removed very slowly from the long sheath with the side-port of the sheath opened to atmosphere and positioned in a dependent position, allowing for slow 'bleeding'. Alternatively, for the larger-diameter sheaths (10F and 12F) in which the dilator does not fit through the detachable hemostatic valve, the dilator is aspirated and flushed slowly while being removed from the long sheath.[7] The adoption of these simple techniques has avoided the introduction of any air into patients.

The device is opened, inspected, and thoroughly soaked in saline solution in order to avoid air embolism. The loader is placed on the delivery cable and the device screwed clockwise onto the delivery cable, ensuring easy unscrewing by several screw–unscrew movements. The device is then pulled into the loader and the detachable hemostatic valve attached to the hub of the loader and used to vigorously flush the device and loader with saline. The loader is then pushed into the hub of the delivery sheath. A 'Luer–Lock' mechanism is present on the larger-diameter sheaths to ensure that they do not separate while the device is being pushed into the delivery sheath. It is helpful to have an assistant hold the loader and delivery sheath together, while the operator pushes the device into the delivery sheath. Alternatively, the fingers of the left hand can be used to stabilize or 'splint' the connection, since 'hang-ups' occasionally occur in this area. The delivery wire is pushed firmly but gently, avoiding rotation and thereby premature unscrewing of the device. This process is performed under fluoroscopic control; additional observation under TEE however is also very useful.

Device-deployment sequence

1. Once the device has reached the distal tip of the sheath, the unit of delivery sheath and cable are pulled back from the left upper pulmonary vein into the middle aspect of the left atrium.
2. The left atrial disk of the device is then pushed out under fluoroscopic and TEE control. Once the disk has conformed fully and is not caught on any adjacent structures, for example, left atrial appendage, mitral valve, pulmonary vein, it is pulled on to the interatrial septum.
3. While maintaining tension on the septum with the left atrial disk, the sheath is withdrawn into the right atrium to release the right atrial disk, which is then gently pushed towards the septum. Though the device initially seems rather bulky, it soon configures into a much flatter profile.[7]
4. Correct device positioning is assessed with TEE and fluoroscopy to ensure that there is no straddling and that the mitral valve and superior vena cava are not encroached upon. Before definitive release of the device, its stability can be tested using 'The Minnesota Wiggle' with, not too vigorous, pulling and pushing of the device on the cable. It is important to realize that prior to release, the whole system is under a significant tension with distortion of structures due to the heavy and stiff delivery cable required to load, introduce, and deploy the device. In many patients the stiffness of the delivery cable applies a straightening force to the device-delivery system after it has been deployed. This can make the device appear to be malaligned with the septum until after the device had been released. However, with experience, this distorting effect can be recognized and the movement of the septum with the device assessed on TEE, while gently pushing and pulling the delivery cable.[7] Release of the device will show an adequate device angulation and profile.

Absent aortic rim and interatrial septal defects with large diameter

Larger defects, particularly those without adequate aortic rim, require a different deployment sequence. Because the left atrial rim size stays at 7 mm for devices measuring 11–32 mm, there is a relatively much smaller device-to-defect ratio with larger devices. During device deployment, the inferior direction of the pullback to the interatrial septum makes it especially likely for the left atrial disk to 'fall through' at the antero-superior (aortic) part, where the septum is particularly deficient. During transesophageal interrogation with the vertical planes, the device may appear to be sitting securely and well deployed; however, the horizontal aortic plane will show the left atrial disk straddling into the right atrium, rather than sitting across the aorta. To avoid this, after opening the left atrial disk, the central waist (or stent) is also developed within the left atrium (a radio-opaque marker on the edge of the right atrial disk indicates when the right atrial disk is about to be deployed). The left atrial disk and waist now have a 'tulip-like' configuration and the waist serves to facilitate self-centering during engagement on to the defect. This maneuver usually proves very helpful. In defects without aortic rim, the device has to splay itself across the aorta (Figure 7.4) and occasionally a device with a slightly larger diameter may have to be implanted in order to have sufficient rim in the left atrial recess beside the aorta.[7]

Other techniques have been described to deal with devices that, although properly sized, keep coming through the defect. The directional Hausdorf-Lock sheath described above is clearly the best approach to aligning the device with the plane of the septum. A long dilator (or ICE catheter) passed from the contralateral femoral vein can be used to prevent the anterior part of the device from prolapsing. A similar approach is to inflate a large occlusion balloon (Meditech, Boston Scientific) alongside the device as it is being deployed and deflate it once the right atrial disk has been deployed.

The device can also be opened towards the right upper pulmonary vein to allow the posterior part of the septum to be abutted by the device before the anterior septum is encountered. Another pulmonary vein maneuver described, is to open the device in the left upper pulmonary vein and then quickly deploy the right atrial disk while the left atrial disk is still hung-up in the pulmonary vein. This technique depends on the length of the constrained device being sufficiently long to keep enough device in the left pulmonary vein while the right atrial disk deploys.

For those defects with a very deficient inferior rim, opening the device in the left upper pulmonary vein may also be helpful. The risk of trauma to the pulmonary vein itself however has to be considered.

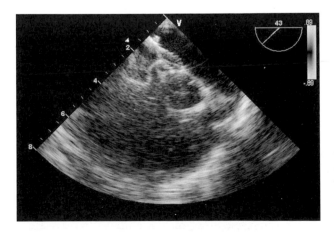

Figure 7.4 Aortic splay. A short axis transesophageal echo cut of the left and right atrial disks of an Amplatzer® septal occluder 'splaying' around the aorta.

Multiple devices

If more than one device is necessary, as in patients with widely separated multiple large defects, the devices are introduced sequentially, using bilateral femoral venous access. It has been our practice to leave the first device attached to the delivery cable until placement of the second device (Figure 7.5). Alternatively, the smaller of the defects can be closed first, then the larger defect crossed and closed through the ipsilateral femoral vein.[7]

Defects associated with atrial septal aneurysms can nearly always be closed with the conventional ASO. This is particularly the case if there is a large defect (usually in the antero-superior area where a PFO would be) associated with the aneurysm (Figure 7.6). It can however be quite time consuming to cross the major defect and requires experienced transesophageal echocardiographic assistance. A Right Judkins catheter and Terumo wire are quite helpful in directing wire passage anteriorly. In a true 'pepper-pot' mutiperforated aneurysmal septum a non-centering cribriform device (AGA Medical) may be deployed in a central defect to eliminate the aneurysm.

Release of the device

Color Doppler imaging reliably demonstrates residual shunts or malalignment; angiography through the side port of the delivery sheath is unnecessary.

With the correct position confirmed, device release is effected by counter-clockwise rotation of the delivery cable using the distally attached pin vise. After release, position and defect closure are assessed with color Doppler imaging and fluoroscopy. Sheath and cable are removed and the puncture sites compressed

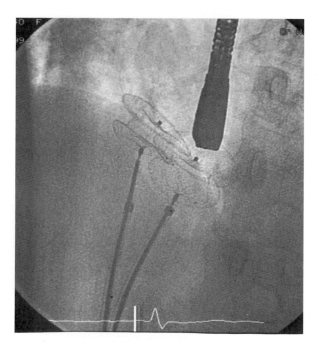

Figure 7.5 Implantation of two devices. Both devices remain attached to their respective delivery cables.

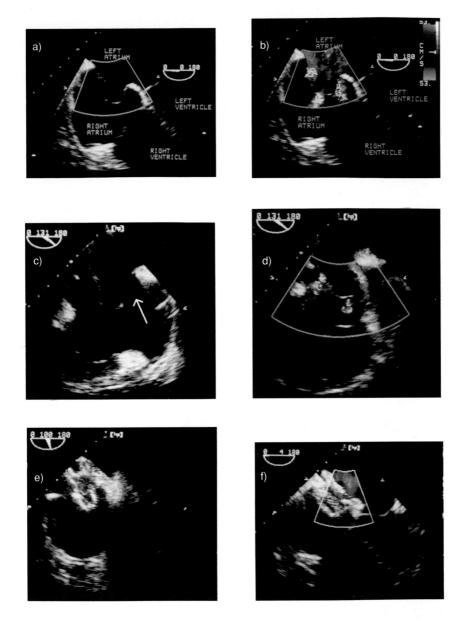

Figure 7.6 Multiperforated interatrial septal aneurysm. Figures 7.6a and b shows a short-axis transesophageal echo cut of an aneurysm of the interatrial septum with multiple perforations and color jets. The largest defect is seen antero-superiorly in a long-axis view as shown in Figures 7.6 c and d. The arrow in Figure 7.6c shows the large antero-superior defect which had to be selectively crossed to implant a device which compressed the aneurysm and occluded all the defects as seen in Figures 7.6e and f.

for at least 15 minutes, avoiding repeated 'check' for cessation of bleeding. A Perclose AT (Abbott Medical) can be used to seal the femoral venous site. We tend to use this in patients who have been taking Plavix or in elderly women who can occasionally develop large hematoma from large venous sheaths. Two further doses of cefuroxime are administered at eight-hourly intervals after recovery from anesthesia.

Complications and procedural difficulties – 'bail out'

Complications are reported to be rare; however, they range from 0 to 11.5% and there is a wide variety owing to operator learning curve and also to the combination of large device and young patient. In our reported patient collective complications consisted, apart from the already mentioned inadvertent air introduction with transient ST-segment changes and the perforation of the left atrial appendage, in overnight migration of a 26 mm device into the pulmonary artery (Figure 7.7), which occurred in an 8-year-old girl. This was discovered on the pre-discharge echocardiographic assessment. The device had to be removed surgically through the tricuspid valve and the ASD was closed with a pericardial patch. The surgeon, however, was able to position the device securely within the defect at the time of surgery, demonstrating that the embolization had occurred due to implantation of the device with the left atrial rim straddling through the antero-superior (aortic) part of the defect. Retrospective analysis of the TEE performed, confirmed this with the color Doppler showing 'color' passing between the left atrial aspect of the device and the aortic root.

Other procedural difficulties encountered have included a 'cobra'-like deformity of the device when extruded. Withdrawal of the device, manual reshaping, and slower reintroduction usually solved this problem. If correct positioning after several attempts does not succeed the device is retrieved and, depending on the underlying problem (such as failure of adequate alignment), replaced with a larger or smaller size or the procedure is abandoned.

The long sheath may kink and/or concertina, particularly if there has been repeated device withdrawal and reintroduction. The operator is then left with a malpositioned device that cannot easily be withdrawn into the sheath. The harder the operator pulls on the cable to get the device back into the sheath, the more the sheath buckles and concertinas. The damaged sheath must be removed and a new one substituted.

A bailout system is available, which allows another delivery cable to be screwed onto the back of the original cable (which remains attached to the malpositioned device). The damaged sheath is then withdrawn and a new specially modified bailout long sheath and dilator (a dilator with a larger lumen to go over the delivery wire) is passed over the extended delivery cable into the patient. This relatively simple process allows the malpositioned device to be withdrawn or repositioned. Using a delivery system at the beginning that is 1 French larger than the recommended sheath system may avoid sheath kinking when the device has to be withdrawn. AGA Medical plan to replace the current range of sheaths with braided kink-resistant sheaths within the next year.

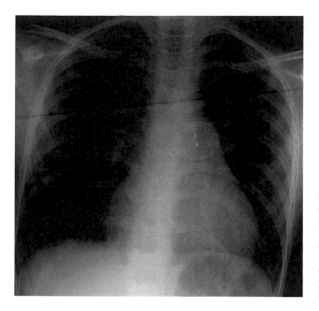

Figure 7.7 Embolized ASD device. A 26 mm Amplatzer® septal occluder has embolized to the pulmonary artery. The device had been implanted without splaying both disks correctly on the aorta in a patient with a deficient aortic rim.

RESULTS

Ideally, the rate of complete closure should be as high as with surgery and the need for re-operation or re-intervention extremely low. After one year the complete occlusion rate with the Amplatzer® device is >90%. Complete closure of the defect occurred in up to 97% of patients at one month and three months post device implantation[13–15] and in 92% to 95% at six months.[6,16,17] The one-year assessment demonstrated complete closure in 93% to 95% of the defects in patients provided with device diameters ranging from 8 to 28 mm,[17,18] showing that the Amplatzer® device produces higher occlusion rates of ASDs with shorter fluoroscopy times. In our patient collective[7] all residual shunts have been small and should not require further intervention. Re-operation was necessary in only one patient with a deformed prototypical device because of a large residual shunt.

Not many long-term follow-up data (>5 years) are available to date; however, one center has observed 151 patients who underwent successful percutaneous closure of ASD between 1995 and 2004, with a follow-up from 56 to 108 months (median 78 months), concluding that the ASO proved to be a safe and effective device for percutaneous closure of ASD II.[19] Another center studied 236 consecutive patients over a period of 4.3 years (median 2.3 years), successfully closing ASDs in 200 patients, with documented complete closure in 94% and trivial residual shunts in 12 patients, concluding efficacy of the ASO with excellent intermediate results.[20]

Several studies compared surgical with transcatheter closure of ASD,[21–23] and despite some limitations in study design (lack of randomization,[21] younger and smaller patients undergoing surgery[22]) all demonstrated substantial advantages of the interventional closure of ASDs with significantly fewer complications, important reduction of hospitalization, reduced need for intensive care (the major area of cost savings to the hospitals)[22] and blood products, less discomfort for the patients, and no incisional scar. However, as one study reminds: 'the surgeon's ability to close any ASD, regardless of anatomy, remains an important advantage of surgery'.[21]

FOLLOW-UP

Aspirin in antiplatelet dose is given once daily and continued for a period of six months. Endocarditis prophylaxis has to be observed during this six-month period. A 12-lead ECG (electrocardiogram), transthoracic echocardiography and chest radiograph are performed after 24 hours. These investigations are repeated at one and three months and again after one and three years. Return to full activity including competitive sports is allowed after four weeks. Magnetic resonance imaging, if required, can be carried out at any time after device implantation.

TECHNIQUE FOR PATENT FORAMEN OVALE CLOSURE

The technique for closure of a patent foramen ovale using an Amplatzer® septal occluder is similar to that for closing an atrial septal defect. The procedure can be done under general anesthetic with transesophageal echocardiographic imaging, or under local anesthetic with intracardiac echocardiographic imaging. Some operators perform this procedure with no periprocedural echocardiography, but merely radiographic imaging. If this latter approach is chosen then it is very important to have excellent and comprehensive transesophageal echocardiography prior to the procedure in order for the defect to have been very well characterized. The first part of the procedure is to cross the patent foramen ovale, which is usually straightforward, but may be technically challenging, particularly if the defect is very small, or if there is a tunnel, which may be difficult to negotiate. A 6 French or 7 French multi-purpose A2 catheter is commonly selected and the oval fossa may be approached either from above or below. One technique is to place the catheter with the curve facing towards the patient's left in the superior vena cava and draw the catheter inferiorly until the tip of the catheter makes a leftwards, sideways movement. The tip of the catheter will then typically lie within the oval fossa and the fossa can be probed. The application of clockwise torque to the catheter may be helpful in the catheter crossing the defect. Alternatively, the catheter may be advanced into the oval fossa from the inferior vena cava and the fossa probed in a similar manner. On occasions the catheter will not pass easily through the foramen ovale, in which case it may be helpful to use a guide-wire. A 0.035 inch J-tipped guide-wire may sufficiently stiffen the tip of the catheter to carry it across. If a Terumo wire is employed then it is very important to be certain where the tip of the catheter lies, as pericardial effusion after the use of this wire in attempting to cross the patent foreman ovale has been recorded. Once the catheter is placed into the left atrium, some operators find it advantageous to take a right upper pulmonary venous angiogram in the left anterior oblique cranial projection, in order to profile the interatrial septum. The catheter is then placed in the left upper pulmonary vein and an exchange length guide-wire positioned with the tip well into the vein. Some operators prefer to use a stiffer guide-wire at this point in order to assist with the next stage of the procedure.

The catheter is withdrawn and if balloon sizing of the patent foramen ovale is to be carried out, then one of two different techniques can be used. Not all operators feel that balloon sizing is required and there is a clear range of opinion as to its role. High-volume users of the Amplatzer® patent foramen ovale occluders often do not use balloon sizing because of the versatility of the devices. Users of the HELEX and STARFlex® devices often do advocate balloon sizing. Balloon sizing can be undertaken using an Amplatzer® balloon in which a sausage-shaped low-pressure balloon is inflated across the defect. An indentation will appear at the site of the atrial septum. The width of the defect can be assessed by radiographic measurement and the operator will get a sense of the length of the defect and whether the anatomy is that of a tunnel.

An alternative method is to use a Boston Meditech sizing balloon, inflated to a certain predetermined amount within the right atrium and then pushed through the septum. The largest size, which will pass through the patent foramen ovale from right to left, gives an estimate of the stretched size of the defect. There are three sizes of specifically designed Amplatzer® patent foramen ovale occluders. Their design is similar to the devices for atrial septal defect closure in that they are made of a double disk Nitinol wire design, but differ in that the devices are not self-centering and have a thin waist made up of the Nitinol wires, rather than a broad waist. The right atrial disk is larger than the left in two of the three sizes and the devices are sized according to the diameter of the right atrial disk. The sizes which are available are 18 mm, 25 mm and 35 mm. For the majority of defects a 25 mm device will be suitable. The 18 mm device has two disks of equal diameter and may be used in children or small adults. The 35 mm device has been advocated for splinting the septum in cases of an atrial septal aneurysm. The devices tend to conform to the anatomy of the PFO and can be used in tunnel anatomy. Some operators have advocated the use of a small atrial septal defect device in cases where balloon sizing shows a diameter of the PFO over 12 mm. The incidence of residual shunting of echo contrast appears less with the use of an ASD occluder for larger-diameter PFOs. Residual shunting of bubbles probably does not matter for the prevention of paradoxical thromboembolism but may be important for prevention of decompression illness in divers.[24]

The technique for delivery of the device is similar to that for an atrial septal defect closure. A delivery sheath with dilator is placed over the wire into the left atrium and then the wire and dilator are carefully removed. The device, preloaded into a short sheath can be advanced into the delivery sheath and the left atrial disk deployed. This disk is then pulled back against the septum and with traction on the system maintained, the sheath can be pulled back so deploying the right atrial disk. It is important to ensure that there is no residual shunt and indeed no coincident atrial septal defect and checks on the stability of the device can be undertaken in the conventional manner. The device is released in a similar manner by unscrewing the loading cable in a counter-clockwise manner.

CONCLUSIONS

The technique of percutaneous ASD closure has evolved enormously over the last decade and the introduction of the Amplatzer® septal occluder has allowed most secundum ASDs in adults and children to be closed percutaneously. Currently no other device is capable of closing large defects. Experience has shown that echocardiographic evaluation of the defect is the most important aspect of the procedure and that the device diameter required to close the defect can often be chosen without recourse to balloon sizing. In fact, balloon sizing is unhelpful in most large and small defects. Maneuvers and special sheaths allow devices to be aligned relatively easily with the septum and help to minimize the size of device required to safely close the defect. Although the very long-term (>10 years) follow-up is not yet available, percutaneous ASD closure has already displaced open-heart surgery as the treatment of choice for secundum atrial septal defects.

REFERENCES

1. Wilmshurst PT, Pearson MJ, Nightingale S, Walsh KP, Morrison WL. Inheritance of persistent foramen ovale and atrial septal defects and the relation to familial migraine with aura. Heart 2004; 90:1315–20.
2. Windecker S, Wahl A, Chatterjee T et al. Percutaneous closure of patent ovale in patients with paradoxical embolism. Circulation 2000; 101:893–8.
3. Martin F, Sanchez PL, Doherty E et al. Percutaneous transcatheter closure of patent foramen ovale in patients with paradoxical embolism. Circulation 2002; 106(9):1121–6.
4. Onorato E, Melzi G, Casilli F et al. Patent foramen ovale with paradoxical embolism: mid-term results of transcatheter closure in 256 patients. J Interv Cardiol 2003; 16(1):43–50.
5. Hamdan MA, Cao Q-L, Hijazi ZM. Amplatzer septal occluder. In Catheter Based Devices for the Treatment of Non-coronary Cardiovascular Disease in Adults and Children. Rao PS, Kern MJ (eds). Philadelphia, Lippincott Williams & Wilkins, 2003; S1–9.
6. Ewert P, Berger F, Daehnert I et al. Transcatheter closure of atrial septal defects without fluoroscopy: feasibility of a new method. Circulation 2000; 101:847–9.
7. Walsh KP, Maadi IM. The Amplatzer septal occluder. Cardiol Young 2000; 10:493–501.
8. Rocchini A, Lock JE. Defect closure: umbrella devices. In Diagnostic and Interventional Catheterization in Congenital Heart Disease, Second Edition. Lock JE, Keane JF, Perry SB (eds). Massachusets, Kluwer Academic Publishers, 2004.
9. Sharafuddin MJA, Gu X, Titus JL et al. Transvenous closure of secundum atrial defects: preliminary results with a new self-expanding Nitinol prosthesis in a swine model. Circulation 1997; 95:2162–8.
10. Rao PS, Langhough R, Beekman RH, Lloyd TR, Sideris EB. Echocardiographic estimation of balloon-stretched diameter of secundum atrial septal defect for transcatheter occlusion. Am Heart J 1992; 124(1):172–5.
11. Castleman AH, Motzkinn SM, Alicandri FP, Bonawit VL. Biocompatibility of nitinol alloy as an implant material. J Biomed Mater Res 1976; 10:695–731.
12. Cragg AH, De Jong SC, Barnhart WH, Landas SK, Smith TP. Nitinol intravascular stent: results of preclinical evaluation. Radiology 1993; 189(3):775–8.
13. Thanopoulos BD, Laskari CV, Tsaousis GS et al. Closure of atrial septal defects with the Amplatzer occlusion device: preliminary results. J Am Coll Cardiol 1998; 31:1110–16.
14. Chan KC, Godman MJ, Walsh K et al. Transcatheter closure of atrial septal defect and interatrial communications with a new self-expanding Nitinol double disc device (Amplatzer septal occluder): multicenter UK experience. Heart 1999; 82:300–6.

15. Fischer G, Kramer HH, Stieh J et al. Transcatheter closure of secundum atrial defects with the new self-centering Amplatzer septal occluder. Eur Heart J 1999; 20:541–9.
16. Hijazi ZM, Cao QL, Patel HT et al. Transcatheter closure of atrial communications (ASD/PFO) in adult patients [CLOSECHEV]18 years of age using the Amplatzer septal occluder: immediate and midterm results. J Am Coll Cardiol 2000; 35(Suppl A):522A.
17. Dhillon R, Thanopoulos B, Tsaousis G et al. Transcatheter closure of atrial septal defects in adults with the Amplatzer septal occluder. Heart 1999; 82:559–62.
18. Walsh KP, Tofeig M, Kitchiner DJ et al. Comparison of the Sideris and Amplatzer septal occlusion devices. Am J Cardiol 1999; 83:933–6.
19. Masura J, Gavora P, Podnar T. Long-term outcome of transcatheter secundum-type atrial septal defect closure using Amplatzer septal occluders. J Am Coll Cardiol 2005; 45:505–7.
20. Fischer G, Stieh J, Uebing A, Hoffmann U, Morf G, Kramer HH. Experience with transcatheter closure of secundum atrial septal defects using the Amplatzer septal occluder: a single centre study in 236 consecutive patients. Heart 2003; 89:199–204.
21. Bialkowski J, Karwot B, Szkutnik M et al. Closure of atrial septal defects in children: surgery versus Amplatzer device implantation. Tex Heart Inst J 2004; 31(3):220–3.
22. Hughes ML, Maskell G, Goh TH, Wilkinson JL. Prospective comparison of costs and short-term health outcomes of surgical versus device closure of atrial septal defect in children. Heart 2002; 88:67–70.
23. Thompson JD, Aburawi EH, Watterson KG, Van Doorn C, Gibbs JL. Surgical and transcatheter (Amplatzer) closure of atrial septal defects: a prospective comparison of results and costs. Heart 2002; 87:466–9.
24. Wilmshurst PT, Nightingale S, Walsh KP, Morrison WL. Effect on migraine of closure of cardiac right-to-left shunts to prevent recurrence of decompression illness or stroke or for hemodynamic reasons. Lancet 2000; 356(9242):1648–51.

8

The Amplatzer* septal occluder

Francisco Garay, Qi-Ling Cao, and Ziyad M Hijazi

Introduction • Selection of patients for device closure • Device description
• Delivery system • Closure procedure • Follow-up • Complications
• Technical tips • Summary

INTRODUCTION

The Amplatzer® septal occluder (ASO) device was designed by Dr Kurt Amplatz
to overcome the limitations of the devices previously used to close atrial septal
defects (ASDs). Those devices had a high incidence of residual shunts; structural
failures due to fractures of their frames; inability to easily retrieve them, and the
need for large delivery systems rendering their use in children limited. The ASO
has become the most desirable device that can be used in both adults and children. It possesses certain characteristics that make it an ideal device for closure
of ASDs including its user-friendly delivery system; high complete closure rate;
small delivery system, and the ability to retrieve or reposition the device prior
to its release from the delivery cable.

The device was first used with good results in an animal model in 1997.[1]
Shortly after, the initial human experience in 30 patients was reported with
encouraging results.[2] Since then, there have been numerous publications from
around the world reporting high efficacy and safety results with this device.[3–6]
In December, 2001, the ASO device received FDA approval for the occlusion of
secundum type ASDs after the positive results of the US multi-center trial that
compared the device results with those obtained by open heart surgery.[7] Since
then, it is estimated that more than 60,000 devices have been implanted worldwide. The international experience using this device has shown immediate
successful closure rates of over 95% that increased to over 99% after one year of
follow-up and to 100% after two years of follow-up.[5,6] Studies comparing ASD
closure using the ASO with that of open heart surgery demonstrated lower
complication rates, shorter length of hospital stay, and reduced costs than the
surgical group.[8–11] There have been three reported cases of device-related deaths
in the literature, a rate much lower than that obtained by open heart surgery.[12]

*Amplazer® is a registered trademark of the AGA Medical Corporation, Golden Valley,
MN.

SELECTION OF PATIENTS FOR DEVICE CLOSURE

The ASO has been designed to close secundum type ASDs; therefore, the use of this device to close primum or sinus venosus type ASDs should not be attempted at all. Usually patients selected for transcatheter ASD closure should have evidence of significant left-to-right shunt, determined either clinically or by the presence of right heart chamber enlargement by transthoracic echocardiography (TTE). In adults, due to the poor echocardiographic windows, a more accurate echocardiographic evaluation is performed using transesophageal echocardiography (TEE). It is necessary to have at least a distance of 5 mm from the margins of the ASD to the mouth of the superior vena cava (SVC), the inferior vena cava (IVC), the posterior wall of the atrium, coronary sinus, the atrioventricular valves, and the right upper pulmonary vein. The anterior rim to the aortic root is frequently deficient and even absent. Its deficiency or absence is not a contraindication to use of the ASO. Contraindications for transcatheter ASD closure using the ASO include: non-reactive obstructive pulmonary vascular disease that can be present in patients over 40 years of age, current systemic or local infection or sepsis within one month of the procedure, bleeding disorders or other contraindications to aspirin therapy, unless other antiplatelet agents such as Clopidogrel can be used for six months, presence of intracardiac thrombus. Nickel allergy is a relative contraindication since this issue has not been clinically significant even in patients with documented nickel allergy. Furthermore, there has not been an increase in blood nickel levels in patients who had Amplatzer® devices implanted.[13]

If a high pulmonary vascular resistance (over 8 Woods units) is found during the catheterization, a trial with pulmonary vasodilators (oxygen 100% and/or inhaled nitric oxide) must be performed, and if pulmonary vascular resistance index remains higher than 6 Woods units, the closure of the defect is contraindicated. In patients older than 65 years of age with large defects, especially if they have another form of cardiac disease (hypertensive, valvular or coronary), it is necessary to evaluate the left ventricle compliance and determine if it will be able to handle the volume overload produced with the ASD closure.[14] This is achieved by measuring the left atrial pressure during balloon occlusion of the defect. We cross the defect with a multi-purpose catheter and position it in the left upper pulmonary vein. An exchange guide-wire is left there and a 27–33 mm Meditech sizing balloon (Boston Scientific Corp., Natick, MA) is used and advanced over the wire until it is in the left atrium. The balloon is inflated and brought tight to the defect to close it. This is documented by echocardiography. Once cessation of shunt occurs, the wire is removed and the left atrial pressure is measured from the distal tip of the balloon. If left atrial pressure increases above 18 mmHg or by more than 5 mmHg from baseline, the procedure is aborted and the patient is sent to the ward for left ventricle conditioning treatment using anticongestive and afterload therapy for 48–72 hours prior to attempting the closure procedure.[15,16] After the conditioning, a repeat cardiac catheterization is performed and the left atrial pressure is measured with temporary balloon occlusion. If the pressure does not exceed 18 mmHg, complete closure is attempted. However, if the left atrial pressure increases to more than 18 mmHg, or by more than 5 mmHg from baseline, a fenestrated ASO device is used.[16]

DEVICE DESCRIPTION

The ASO is a self-centering device with a double disk conformation, constructed from a 0.004–0.0075 inch Nitinol wire mesh. Nitinol is an alloy (55% nickel and 45% titanium) that has super elastic properties; it provides shape memory permitting the device to be loaded straight into a delivery sheath and then recover its conformation when deployed across the ASD (Figure 8.1). The device has a 3–4 mm connecting waist between the two disks. The device size is determined by the diameter of this connecting waist. The device is available in sizes ranging from 4 to 40 mm (one mm increment from 4–20 mm devices and 2 mm increments from 20 to 40 mm devices). The two flat disks extend radially beyond the connecting waist to secure the anchorage. The left atrial disk is larger than the right atrial disk due to the usual left-to-right shunt seen in ASD. For devices ranging from 4–10 mm in diameter, the left disk is 12 mm and the right disk is 8 mm larger than the waist. For devices ranging from 11–34 mm in diameter, the left disk is 14 mm and the right disk is 10 mm larger than the waist. For devices larger than 34 mm, the left disk is 16 mm and the right disk is 10 mm larger than the connecting waist. Dacron polyester patches are sewn into each disk and the connecting waist to increase thrombogenicity of the device. A stainless steel sleeve with a female thread is laser-welded to the right disk. This is used to screw the delivery cable to the device, so it is a security mechanism that permits the device to be repositioned even after both disks have been deployed.

DELIVERY SYSTEM

The Amplatzer® delivery system is supplied separate from the device and contains a long delivery sheath with its dilator, a loading device, a delivery cable, and a plastic pin vise.

The delivery sheath is available in sizes from 6 to 12Fr and has a 45° angled tip. The 6Fr sheath has a length of 60 cm, the 7Fr sheath is available in lengths of 60 and 80 cm and the 8, 9, 10 and 12Fr sheaths are all 80 cm long. The loading device is used to collapse the device in a straight fashion to be introduced into the delivery sheath. The delivery cable (0.081 inch) is screwed to the device and allows loading, placement, and retrieval of the device. The plastic pin vise facilitates unscrewing of the delivery cable from the device after the deployment.

It is recommended to use a 6Fr delivery system for devices less than 10 mm in diameter; a 7Fr sheath for devices 10–15 mm; an 8Fr delivery system for devices

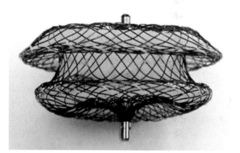

Figure 8.1 The Amplatzer® Septal Occluder with two disks and a connecting waist.

16–19 mm; a 9Fr sheath for devices 20–26 mm; a 10Fr delivery system for devices 28–34 mm, and a 12Fr sheath for the 36, 38, and 40 mm devices. However, to facilitate capturing of the devices, we suggest upsizing by 1Fr from the recommended delivery sheath size.

CLOSURE PROCEDURE

All previous data related to the patient and the defect to be closed need to be previously reviewed, availability of appropriate devices and delivery systems needs to be ensured, as well as all materials eventually necessary to the success of the procedure.[17,18] A failed procedure due to lack of appropriate equipments is inexcusable! Aspirin 81–325 mg daily should be started 48 hours prior to the procedure to reduce the risk of early thrombus formation after the procedure. Alternatively, Clopidogrel 75 mg could be used.

Patients are usually placed under general anesthesia if TEE is used to guide the procedure. Recently intracardiac echocardiography (ICE) has permitted the procedure to be performed under conscious sedation avoiding the risks and costs of general anesthesia.[19–21] Routine left and right heart catheterization is performed to measure pulmonary artery pressure, and to calculate the left-to-right shunt and the pulmonary vascular resistance. The right femoral vein is accessed via two separate punctures: an 8Fr sheath for the cardiac catheterization and device delivery and an 8 or 11Fr sheath for the ICE catheter. We usually do not access the femoral artery if ICE is used; however, we recommend an arterial access be obtained if the procedure is done under TEE and general anesthesia. For ICE, we have been using the 8 or 10Fr shaft AcuNav catheter (Acuson, A Siemens company, Mountain View, CA). If femoral venous access is not available, it is preferable to use the transhepatic approach. Delivery of the device from the jugular or subclavian veins is difficult. Heparin is administered to maintain an activated clotting time (ACT) above 200 seconds at the time of device deployment (children: 100 U/kg, adults: 3000–5000 Units). Antibiotic coverage is recommended for the procedure (Cefazolin; children: 25 mg/kg/dose, adults: 1 g iv/dose), the first dose at the time of the procedure and two additional doses 6–8 hours apart.

Anatomic characterization of the defect (location, size, additional defects, and surrounding rims) is necessary prior to device delivery. This can be achieved by TEE or ICE.[19,20] Superior and inferior rims are better seen in the bicaval view (long axis), the posterior and anterior rims are better evaluated in the short axis view. All steps to deliver and deploy the device are guided by echocardiography and fluoroscopy (Figures 8.2 and 8.3).

A multipurpose or an angiographic catheter is advanced through the defect into the right upper pulmonary vein and angiography is performed in the hepatoclavicular projection (35° LAO/35° cranial) to delineate the entire length and shape of the atrial septum and location of the ASD (Figure 8.3). This image will be useful later to evaluate the device position as seen in the same projection prior to its release from the cable. Then an extra stiff exchange length guide-wire is positioned in the left upper pulmonary vein. We usually use Amplatzer® Super Stiff Exchange Guide wire 0.035 inch with 1 cm floppy tip, but any extra stiff J-tipped wire could be used. A sizing balloon catheter is advanced over this wire across the ASD, this is optional but recommended. We use the Amplatzer® sizing

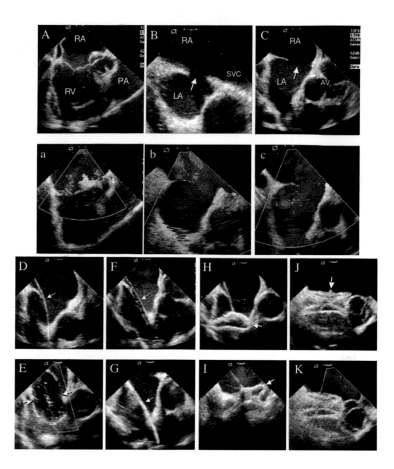

Figure 8.2 Intracardiac echocardiographic images in a 51-year-old female with severe scoliosis and large secundum ASD. **A, a** Home view without and with color Doppler demonstrating the right atrium, tricuspid valve, right ventricle, aortic root, and pulmonary artery. **B, b** Caval view without and with color Doppler demonstrating the entire superior rim and the defect (arrow). **C, c** Short axis view demonstrating the defect (arrow), aortic root, absent anterior rim and good posterior rim and both atria. **D** The exchange wire (arrow) across the defect into the left upper pulmonary vein. **E** Sizing balloon through the defect to obtain the 'stop flow' diameter (arrows) of the defect to be 32 mm. **F** Delivery sheath (arrow) across the defect into the left upper pulmonary vein. **G** The device (34 mm Amplatzer®) is being pushed inside the delivery system. **H** The left atrial disk (arrow) deployed in the left atrium. **I** The right atrial disk (arrow) deployed in the right atrium. **J** The device (arrow) released demonstrating good position in the short axis view. **K** Color Doppler demonstrating no residual shunt. RA: right atrium; LA: left atrium; RV: right ventricle; AV: aortic valve; PA: pulmonary artery; SVC: superior vena cava.

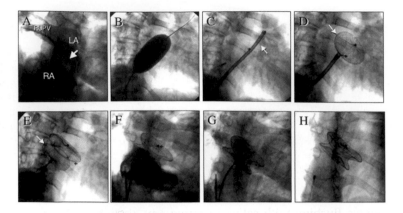

Figure 8.3   Cine angiographic images in the same patient as Figure 8.2. **A** Angiogram in the right upper pulmonary vein in the hepatoclavicular projection (35° LAO/35° cranial) demonstrating left-to-right shunt (arrow). **B** Cine image during balloon sizing of the defect demonstrating the 'stop flow' diameter of the defect;. **C** Cine fluoroscopy during advancement of the device inside the delivery sheath (white arrow). **D** Cine fluoroscopy during deployment of the left atrial disk of the 34 mm Amplatzer® device (white arrow). **E** Cine fluoroscopy during deployment of the right atrial disk (white arrow). **F** Angiogram in the right atrium demonstrating opacification of the right atrial disk only. **G** Cine angiography of the pulmonary levophase of a right atrial angiogram prior to device release demonstrating good device position. **H** Cine fluoroscopy after the device has been released demonstrating good device position.

balloon that is a double lumen balloon catheter with a 7Fr shaft size. This balloon is 45° angled and has radio-opaque markers for calibration at 2, 5, and 10 mm (inner to inner marker). It comes in two sizes: 24 mm (maximum volume is 30 ml for sizing defects up to 22 mm) and 34 mm (maximum volume is 90 ml for sizing defects up to 40 mm). We prefer to use the 34 mm sizing balloon which we directly introduce through the skin. The balloon is made from nylon and is very compliant making it ideal for sizing ASD by flow occlusion and preventing overstretching of the defect. Alternatively, the NuMED sizing balloon catheters (NuMED Inc., Hopkinton, NY) can be used for sizing. They are available in various sizes (20–40 mm and various lengths 3–5 cm). It is important to perform carefully the stop flow technique. For this the balloon is placed across the defect under fluoroscopic and echocardiographic guidance and then inflated with diluted contrast until the left-to-right shunt ceases (stop flow technique) as observed by color flow Doppler on TEE or ICE (Figures 8.2E and 8.3B). The indentations in the balloon made by the margins of the ASD are measured on echocardiographic (long axis view) or fluoroscopic images (beam perpendicular to the balloon). Usually the echocardiographic measurements are more reliable than the fluoroscopic measurements. The device used is usually selected to be 1–2 mm larger than the diameter of the balloon when cessation of flow occurred during sizing of the defect. If the 'stop flow' diameter of the defect is more than 50% of the two-dimensional diameter by TEE/ICE, one should question this measurement and perhaps repeat the sizing. Alternatively, a device 20–25%

larger than the two-dimensional diameter of the defect by TEE/ICE is chosen for the closure.

Once the device size has been chosen, the sizing balloon is removed and an appropriate delivery sheath is advanced over the super stiff guide-wire. Once the dilator reaches the right atrium, the delivery sheath by itself is advanced over the wire and dilator until the tip of the sheath is in the left upper pulmonary vein (Figure 8.3C). This is done to reduce the risk of introduction of air into the system. Once the tip of the sheath is in the left upper pulmonary vein, the dilator and wire are removed as one unit while the hub of the sheath is between and lower than the patient's legs. From our experience, this technique avoids or minimizes any air introduction.

The delivery cable is screwed to the selected device and withdrawn into the loader under saline seal. A Touhy-Borst Y connector previously attached to the loader allows flushing with saline to purge any air bubble. Next, the loader containing the device is attached to the proximal hub of the delivery sheath, and the device is advanced to the distal tip of the sheath, taking care not to rotate the cable while advancing it in the long sheath to prevent premature unscrewing of the device. Then, the cable and delivery sheath are pulled back as one unit out of the pulmonary vein into the middle of the left atrium. Pulling back the sheath while maintaining the cable position deploys the left atrial disk (Figures 8.2H and 8.3D). Part of the connecting waist should be deployed in the left atrium very close to the atrial septum. Finally, withdrawing the delivery sheath off the cable, the connecting waist and the right atrial disk are deployed in the ASD itself and in the right atrium respectively (Figures 8.2I and 8.3E).

In cases of multiple ASDs, a number of considerations are important.[18,22,23] An accurate echocardiographic evaluation of the atrial septum is needed, focusing on number and size of defects, distance between them, surrounding rims, and presence of aneurysmal septum. If more than 7 mm rim of tissue separates the two defects, two separate catheters are placed across each defect. Color Doppler is applied to the entire septum during balloon sizing of each defect to assess the presence of other defects. The 'stop flow diameter' of each defect is then measured by echocardiography (TEE/ICE). The smaller device is deployed but not released, then the larger device is deployed. The devices are released sequentially starting with the smaller device. The two devices may overlap (the larger device sandwiching the smaller one) resulting in a slightly larger profile; however, this has not resulted in any clinical problem on follow up. If the defects are small and close to each other (multifenestrated), one could attempt the closure using the appropriate-sized Cribriform device. The Cribriform device is available in three sizes: 18, 25, and 35 mm with both disks equal in size.

The proper device position on the atrial septum is assessed by fluoroscopy and TEE/ICE images. Fluoroscopy in the hepatoclavicular projection must show both disks parallel to each other and separated from each other by the atrial septum (Figure 8.3F). A gentle push forward and pull backward (Minnesota wiggle) of the cable while fixing the sheath will test stability of the device (this is evaluated under fluoroscopy and echocardiography). Optional angiography of the right atrium using the side arm of the delivery sheath can be performed in this projection. The proper position of the device manifests by opacification of the right atrial disk alone when the contrast is in the right atrium (Figure 8.3F) and the opacification of the left atrial disk alone on pulmonary levophase

(Figure 8.3G). In addition the echocardiogram (TEE/ICE) must demonstrate the presence of one disk in each atrial chamber. Color Doppler evaluation over the device usually shows a small color signal between the two disks (foaming) that represents blood flow across the device mesh and usually disappears within the first 24 hours. If the position is uncertain or questionable after all these maneuvers, the device can be recaptured and repositioned following similar steps. After the position of the device has been verified, the device is released by counterclockwise rotation of the delivery cable using the pin vise. Immediately after the device has been released, the delivery cable is pulled back into the sheath and out of the body. The sheath is pulled back into the IVC. Assessment of the final result of the closure procedure is performed immediately with TEE or ICE (Figures 8.2J and 8.2K). At the end of the procedure, ACT is rechecked and the sheath is removed. If the ACT is higher than 250 seconds, we reverse the effects of heparin with protamine sulfate. If the procedure is performed with endotracheal intubation, extubation of the patient is performed in the catheterization lab.

FOLLOW-UP

Patients must stay overnight in a telemetry ward to observe for arrhythmias. The following day, an ECG, chest X-ray, and a TTE with color Doppler evaluation are performed to evaluate the position of the device and the presence of residual shunt, also to look for any potential complications. If the closure is complete, the next visit can be after six months. However, if there is residual shunt, a visit can be scheduled after one month. Then annual visits may be scheduled to monitor the device and the rare possibility of device erosion. Long-term follow-up must include ECG and/or 24-hour ambulatory ECG monitoring. Any symptom including chest pain, shortness of breath or syncope should be followed-up immediately with an echocardiogram to rule out pericardial effusion due to device erosion.

Patients are asked to take aspirin 81–325 mg orally once daily for six months, and endocarditis prophylaxis when necessary for six months after the procedure. If complete closure is documented at the six-month visit, endocarditis prophylaxis and aspirin are discontinued. Complete neoendothelialization and fibrous incorporation of the device has been reported at three months after the procedure.[1] Full activity including competitive and contact sports are restricted after the procedure to minimize the infrequent risk of late embolization. This restriction is variable around 4–8 weeks depending on the size of the defect and sufficiency of its rims.[24]

COMPLICATIONS

Air embolism

Meticulous technique should be used to prevent air entry into the left side that may result in coronary ischemia and stroke. Free flow of blood out of the sheath when it is at the mouth of the left upper pulmonary vein must be allowed, avoiding forceful negative pressure to aspirate it. If a large amount of air is introduced in the left atrium it will usually pool in the right coronary sinus and right coronary artery. This can produce bradycardia, profound hypotension or asystole. If this occurs, immediately place a right coronary catheter in the right coronary sinus and forcefully inject saline or contrast to displace the air and reperfuse the right coronary system.

Cobra-head formation

This occurs when the LA disk develops an abnormal profile when deployed, mimicking a cobra head. This usually occurs when the LA disk is inadvertently opened in the pulmonary vein or LA appendage, when the LA is too small to accommodate the device or it was loaded with an unusual strain. In this situation check the site of deployment or recapture the device, remove it to inspect and reintroduce it. If the cobra-head forms outside the body, use a different device and send back the device to the manufacturer for inspection. Never release a device if the left disk has a cobra-head appearance.

Device embolization

This can occur during the procedure, especially if the rims are insufficient to support the device or due to an inadvertent prolapse of part of the device across the septum before releasing it. If embolization occurs, the device must be removed either surgically or by transcatheter snare techniques. Snaring is difficult and requires an experienced operator in snaring techniques. A long Mullins sheath 2Fr sizes larger than the sheath used to deliver the device is needed. We use the Amplatzer® goose-neck snare (ev3, Plymouth, MN). One should avoid pulling the device across valves, since it may damage the chordae and leaflets. On rare occasions, if the left atrial disk can not be collapsed inside the sheath, another snare is introduced from the right internal jugular vein to snare the stud of the microscrew of the left atrial disk and stretch it towards the internal jugular vein while an assistant pulls the device with snare towards the femoral vein. This permits the device to collapse further and come out of the sheath in the femoral vein. Late non-procedural embolization has been reported and this has motivated the restriction of physical activity after the procedure for at least four weeks.[24]

Arrhythmias

An increase in atrial arrhythmias occurs following the procedure, but this is a transient phenomenon that resolves within six months.[25,26] Transient AV block has rarely been reported (1–5%) and there only has been one reported case in the literature requiring pacemaker implantation.[25,27] It has been suggested that AV conduction abnormalities can be related to the device size, which just emphasizes the importance of avoiding placement of an oversized device. If atrioventricular block occurs during the procedure, one should remove the device and attempt with a smaller device.

Cardiac perforation and tamponade

Cardiac perforation and tamponade are extremely infrequent (<0.1 %). As of September 2005, there have been a total of 36 cases of erosion reported to the manufacturer of the device with a total of four deaths (two deaths were definitely not device related, but procedure related [perforation of the right upper pulmonary vein with the dilator and perforation of the left atrial appendage with a wire]). It is estimated that as of that date, a total of 60,000 implants had been performed worldwide with the ASO, giving an incidence of 0.06%. Most of these erosions occurred within the first 24 to 48 hours; however, cases have been reported as late as three years from implantation. This has been consistently reported to occur at the dome of the atria, near the aortic root and related to defects with deficient anterior/superior rims.[12,28] The mechanism seems to be erosion of the free atrial wall adjacent to the atrial septum by the edges of the device, producing pericardial effusion. The close proximity of the aorta to the anterior and superior rim of the defect may make the aorta vulnerable to erosion once the device has eroded the atrial wall, producing aortic to atrial fistula.[29] To minimize this risk, one should not implant an oversized device (not more than 30% of the two-dimensional diameter of the defect) and use the 'stop flow' technique when balloon sizing. All patients must be observed overnight in the hospital after the procedure and an echocardiographic evaluation of the device and heart is performed prior to discharge. Any amount of pericardial effusion that is more than baseline or symptoms of chest pain or shortness of breath should prompt further clinical evaluation and another echocardiographic evaluation within 12 hours. In addition to the erosion caused by the device, perforations of the pulmonary veins and left atrial appendage by the wires or catheters have been reported causing pericardial effusion, emphasizing the importance of meticulous techniques while performing such procedures.[12]

Headaches/migraines

Approximately 5–10% of patients who undergo device closure of their defects suffer from headaches and migraine with aura. Extensive evaluation of such patients has not revealed any specific causes. When such patients present (usually within the first few weeks from closure), a TTE should be performed to rule out the presence of any macroscopic clots on the device. If there are neurologic findings, a CT scan or MRI should also be done. If all tests are negative, we have been treating such patients with 75 mg Clopidogrel for 1–3 months in addition to the aspirin. In most patients, these symptoms disappear within a few days of treatment.

TECHNICAL TIPS

Prolapse of the left atrial disk

This can occur during the deployment especially in patients with large defects and deficient anterior/superior rims. In this situation the left atrial disk deploys perpendicular to the septum; due to the deficient anterior/superior rim, the left atrial disk prolapses through the defect to the right atrium. Different techniques have been described to prevent prolapse of the disk and to facilitate transcatheter closure of large defects. The deployment of the device in the right or left upper pulmonary veins rather than the left atrium followed by release of the waist and right atrial disk in a rapid sequence helps to keep the device parallel to the atrial septum.[30] An alternative technique that we find very helpful is the use of a specially designed long sheath with stiffer, sharper posterior curves (Hausdorf Sheath, Cook Inc., Bloomington, IN). This sheath is available in sizes ranging from 10–12Fr. Another technique that has been reported is the use of the long dilator of the delivery sheath from the contralateral femoral vein to hold the left atrial disk in the left atrium while deploying the waist and right atrial disk in their respective locations.[31] Similarly a balloon catheter can be used to hold the left atrial disk during deployment of the waist and right atrial disk, in a way similar to the dilator technique.[32] Finally, the last technique is to deploy the device over a wire anchored in the left upper pulmonary vein. This would require passage of the guide-wire in the middle of the connecting waist and each disk. Once both disks are deployed in their respective locations, the wire is removed and the device is released.

Accordion effect of the delivery sheath

Attempts to recapture the device can produce damage to the delivery sheath. In this situation the Amplatzer® Exchange (Rescue) System can be used. This has the same components as the regular delivery system with the dilator having a larger internal lumen diameter (0.088 inch) allowing the dilator to pass over the cable. If an implanted device cannot be recaptured, one should connect the cable from the rescue system to the end of the cable attached to the device at its proximal end outside the body, thus making it an exchange length cable. The sheath is removed and the new delivery sheath with its special dilator are advanced over the cable. The device then can be easily recaptured. The rescue system is available in 9 and 12Fr sizes. We recommend using the 9Fr system for devices up to 24 mm and the 12Fr system for devices larger than 24 mm.

SUMMARY

The ASO device has demonstrated excellent clinical success in closing ASDs. The immediate success rate is greater than 97%, and our experience suggests that, with proper device selection and placement, 100% closure can be obtained. The ASO has proven to be safe and user-friendly. The reproducibility of these results has been high by different groups. Therefore, we believe the Amplatzer® septal occluder device is the best available option for treatment of suitable secundum type ASDs. The clinical results are very encouraging with a steep learning curve. Even closure of large defects with deficient rims is possible.[18,33]

REFERENCES

1. Sharafuddin M, Gu X, Titus J et al. Transvenous closure of secundum atrial defects. Preliminary results with a new self-expanding nitinol prosthesis in a swine model. Circulation 1997; 95(8):2162–8.
2. Masura J, Gavora P, Formatek A et al. Transcatheter closure of secundum atrial defects using the new self-centering Amplatzer septal occluder: Initial human experience. Cathet Cardiovasc Diagn 1997; 42(4):388–93.
3. Thanopoulos B, Lskari C, Tsaousis G et al. Closure of atrial septal defects with the Amplatzer occlusion device: Preliminary results. J Am Coll Cardiol 1998; 31(5):1110–16.

4. Chan K, Godman M, Walsh K et al. Transcatheter closure of atrial septal defect and interatrial communications with a new self expanding nitinol double disk device (Amplatzer septal occluder): multicentre UK experience. Heart 1999; 82(3):300–6.
5. Omeish A, Hijazi ZM. Transcatheter closure of atrial septal defects in children and adults using the Amplatzer Septal Occluder. J Interven Cardiol 2001; 14(1):37–44.
6. Yew G, Wilson N. Transcatheter atrial septal defect closure with the Amplatzer Septal Occluder: Five-year follow-up. Catheter Cardiovasc Interv 2005; 64(2):193–6.
7. Hijazi ZM, Radtke W, Ebeid M et al. Trascatheter closure of atrial septal defects using Amplatzer septal occluder: Results of phase II US multicenter trial. (abstract). Circulation 1999; 100(18,Suppl 1):I-804.
8. Berger F, Vogel M, Alexi-Meskishvili V et al. Comparison of results and complications of surgical and Amplatzer device closure of atrial septal defects. J Thorac Cardiovasc Surg 1999; 118(4):674–8.
9. Bialkowski J, Karwot B, Szkutnik M et al. Closure of atrial septal defects in children: surgery versus Amplatzer device implantation. Tex Heart Inst J 2004; 31(3):220–3.
10. Du ZD, Hijazi ZM, Kleinman CS et al. Comparison between transcatheter and surgical closure of secundum atrial septal defect in children and adults: results of a multicenter nonrandomized trial. J Am Coll Cardiol 2002; 39(11):1836–44.
11. Kim J, Hijazi ZM. Clinical outcomes and costs of Amplatzer transcatheter closure as compared with surgical closure of ostium secundum atrial septal defects. Med Sci Monit 2002; 8(12):CR787–91.
12. Amin Z, Hijazi ZM, Bass J et al. Erosion of Amplatzer septal occluder device after closure of secundum atrial septal defects: Review of registry of complications and recommendations to minimize future risk. Catheter Cardiovasc Interv 2004; 63(4):496–502.
13. Kong H, Wilkinson JL, Coe JY et al. Corrosive behaviour of Amplatzer devices in experimental and biological environments. Cardiol Young 2002; 12(3):260–5.
14. Ewert P, Berger F, Nagdyman N. Masked left ventricular restriction in elderly patients with atrial septal defects: a contraindication for closure? Catheter Cardiovasc Interv 2001; 52(2):177–80.
15. Schubert S, Peters B, Abdul-Khaliq H et al. Left ventricular conditioning in the elderly patient to prevent congestive heart failure after transcatheter closure of atrial septal defect. Catheter Cardiovasc Interv 2005; 64(3):333–7.
16. Holzer R, Cao QL, Hijazi ZM. Closure of a moderately large atrial septal defect with a self-fabricated fenestrated Amplatzer septal occluder in an 85–year-old patient with reduced diastolic elasticity of the left ventricle. Catheter Cardiovasc Interv 2005; 64(4):513–18
17. Waigh D, Koenig P, Cao QL et al. Transcatheter closure of secundum atrial septal defects using the Amplatzer septal occluder: Clinical experience and technical considerations. Curr Intervent Cardiol Rep 2000; 2(1):70–7.
18. Harper R, Mottram P, McGaw D. Closure of secundum atrial septal defects with the Amplatzer septal occluder device: techniques and problems. Cathet Cardiovasc Intervent 2002; 57(4):508–24.
19. Hijazi ZM, Wang Z, Cao Q, Koenig P, Waight D, Lang R. Transcatheter closure of atrial septal defects and patent foramen ovale under intracardiac echocardiographic guidance: feasibility and comparison with transesophageal echocardiography. Cathet Cardiovasc Intervent 2000; 52(2):194–9.
20. Koenig P, Cao QL, Heitschmidt M, Waight DJ, Hijazi ZM. Role of intracardiac echocardiographic guidance in transcatheter closure of atrial septal defects and patent foramen ovale using the Amplatzer device. J Interv Cardiol 2003; 16(1):51–62.
21. Alboliras ET, Hijazi ZM. Comparison of costs of intracardiac echocardiography and transesophageal echocardiography in monitoring percutaneous device closure of atrial septal defect in children and adults. Am J Cardiol 2004; 94(5):690–2.
22. Cao QL, Radtke W, Berger F, Zhu W, Hijazi ZM. Transcatheter closure of multiple atrial septal defects. Initials results and value of two- and three-dimensional transesophageal echocardiography. Eur Heart J 2000; 21(11):941–7.

23. Szkutnik M, Masura J, Bialkowski J et al. Transcatheter closure of double atrial septal defects with a single Amplatzer device. Catheter Cardiovasc Interv 2004; 61(2):237–41.
24. Mashman W, King S, Jacobs W, Ballard W. Two cases of late embolization of Amplatzer septal occluder devices to the pulmonary artery following closure of secundum atrial septal defects. Cathet Cardiovasc Intervent 2005; 65(4):588–92.
25. Hill S, Berul C, Patel H et al. Early ECG abnormalities associated with transcatheter closure of atrial septal defects using the Amplatzer septal occluder. J Interv Card Electrophysiol 2000; 4(3):469–74.
26. Hessling G, Hyca S, Brockmeier K, Ulmer HE. Cardiac dysrhythmias in pediatric patients before and 1 year after transcatheter closure of atrial septal defects using the amplatzer septal occluder. Pediatr Cardiol 2003; 24(3):259–62. Epub 2003 Jan 15.
27. Suda K, Raboisson MJ, Piette E, Dahdah NS, Miro J. Reversible atrioventricular block associated with closure of atrial septal defects using the Amplatzer device. J Am Coll Cardiol 2004; 43(9):1677–82.
28. Divekar A, Gaamangwe T, Shaikh N, Raabe M, Ducas J. Cardiac perforation after device closure of atrial septal defects with the Amplatzer septal occluder. J Am Coll Cardiol 2005; 45(8):1213–18.
29. Chun D, Turrentine M, Moustapha A, Hoyer M. Development of aorta-to-right atrial fistula following closure of secundum atrial septal defect using the Amplatzer septal occluder. Catheter Cardiovasc Interv 2003; 58(2):246–51.
30. Varma C, Benson LN, Silversides C et al. Outcomes and alternative techniques for device closure of the large secundum atrial septal defect. Catheter Cardiovasc Interv 2004; 61:131–9.
31. Wahab H, Bairam A, Cao Q et al. Novel technique to prevent prolapse of the Amplatzer Septal Occluder through large atrial septal defect. Catheter Cardiovasc Interv 2003; 60(4):543–545.
32. Dalvi B, Pinto R, Gupta A. new technique for device closure of large atrial septal defects. Catheter Cardiovasc Interv 2005; 64(1):102–7.
33. Berger F, Ewert P, Abdul-Khaliq H et al. Percutaneous closure of large atrial septal defects with the Amplatzer septal occluder: technical overkill or recommendable alternative treatment? J Interv Cardiol 2001; 14(1):63–7.

9

Interventional closure of defects in the atrial septum using the HELEX septal occluder

Neil Wilson

Introduction • **ASD closure** • **Patent foramen ovale closure** • **Closure of fenestrated fontan** • **Problems, risks, complications** • **Conclusions**

INTRODUCTION

The HELEX device is a non-self-centering double disk device of Nitinol and ePTFE (Figure 9.1). The device is designed such that, following introduction across the septum, one disk is constituted on the left atrial side and the other on the right atrial side of the septum. The construction of the device consists of a curtain of ePTFE (Goretex™, WL Gore & Associates Flagstaff, Arizona, USA) bonded to a single-piece wire frame of Nitinol 0.012 inches. The Nitinol is prepared in the manner of a helical pattern of opposing rotations which on full configuration assumes two parallel disks. The device is delivered through its own composite triaxial 10Fr delivery catheter with a workable length of 75 cm. This obviates the need for a long trans-septal sheath. For patent foramen ovale the delivery system can be monorailed through a hole close to its distal end using a wire placed through a diagnostic catheter positioned in one of the left pulmonary veins.

The device is available in 15, 20, 25, 30 and 35 mm diameters. The devices are delivered through a short 10Fr femoral vein sheath, though if using the monorail technique a short 12Fr femoral sheath is required.

The HELEX device is designed to be flexible and atraumatic, molding itself to the atrial septum and contiguous structures, rendering it particularly appealing for use in a growing heart. Similarly the proven low thrombogenicity of ePTFE imparts confidence in delivering devices on the systemic side of the circulation (left atrium). This is of particular relevance in closure of the patent foramen ovale (PFO) where there are implications of thrombotic events to the systemic circulation, producing transient ischemic attacks and strokes. ePTFE has been used in various formats as patches and vascular tubes in the growing heart for almost 30 years now, and thus has proven longevity and biocompatibility with rapid endothelialization characteristics. Studies particular to the HELEX device have confirmed this excellent biocompatibility[1] (Figure 9.2).

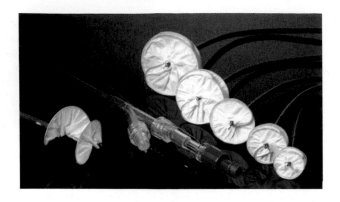

Figure 9.1 Range of HELEX devices from 15–35 mm in 5 mm increments. Also pictured is the integral 10Fr delivery catheter system.

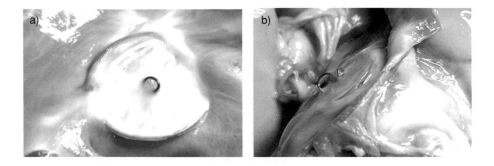

Figure 9.2 HELEX explant from animal compatibility studies. a) Left atrial aspect showing distal eyelet. b) Right atrial aspect with lock mechanism evident. There is virtually complete endothelialization in this specimen three months following implantation. The surface of the device is largely incorprated into the surrounding native atrial tissue.

ASD CLOSURE

Patient selection

The HELEX occluder is designed to occlude central (secundum) type atrial septal defects (ASDs).[2] In keeping with other available occlusion devices, patients with sinus venosus defects and primum defects are not suitable for interventional closure with the HELEX device. The morphology of secundum atrial septal defects is, of course, variable and multiple defects,[3] fenestrated,[4] and aneurysmal defects can be closed[5] using this device. A deficient anterior superior rim, where there is a lack of effacement of the atrial septum at the aorta, can also be accommodated by relative oversizing of the device. In most patients the clinical indication for closure is volume loading of the right ventricle, with right ventricular diastolic dimensions measured on an M Mode echocardiogram in excess of two standard deviations from the mean. The long-term sequelae of right heart dilation and increased pulmonary blood flow have been discussed. Sometimes, patients with a small ASD and normal cardiac dimensions are referred for ASD closure because of symptoms and signs of thromboembolic events. Such indications are more commonly associated with patent foramen ovale.

A non-self-centering device up to defect diameter ratio of 1.8–2.0 is recommended for atrial septal defects. With the largest available device being 35 mm, the largest diameter defect closable would be in the region of 18–19 mm. There is a proviso, however, in that children with large ASDs have a relatively small left atrium, experience has shown that the 30 and 35 mm devices do not sit effectively on the left atrial side of the septum in children weighing less than 25 kg. For most operators precardiac catheter assessment is usually using transthoracic echocardiography. It is likely, therefore, that defects measuring more than 15 mm on a standard transthoracic echocardiogram will balloon size to 18 mm or more and be unsuitable for a HELEX device.

Technique

A fairly standard technique of implantation is employed. In children general anesthesia is required usually with endotracheal intubation. Simultaneous multiplane transesophageal echocardiography is commenced and the morphology of the ASD with respect to size, margins, proximity to the aorta, and atrioventricular valves is assessed. At this stage, multiple defects, not apparent on transthoracic echo may be imaged, as well as fenestrations and aneurysms of the septum. Venous access is established through the right femoral vein with a short (15–20 cm) 10Fr gauge valved sheath. Invasive arterial pressure monitoring is not required. In the presence of a dilated right heart it is not my usual practice to perform a diagnostic type hemodynamic/saturation study. Under general anesthetic even with low inspired oxygen concentration, most patients are supersaturated and the modified Fick method produces inaccurate shunt calculation.

Heparin 100 U/kg is administered intravenously and a diagnostic multipurpose catheter advanced from the inferior vena cava through the right atrium to the left atrium and, by choice, usually the left upper pulmonary vein. This maneuver is entirely to facilitate positioning of a heavy duty type 0.035 inch guide-wire which will subsequently support a sizing balloon. There are currently three types of sizing balloon: the PTS has its calibration marks on the shaft of the catheter within the balloon. It is important, therefore, that a dilute contrast mixture of one part contrast to three parts saline be used for balloon inflation otherwise it is not possible to identify the calibration markers on fluoroscopy. The second, AGA, angled catheter has its markers on the catheter shaft proximal to the balloon, overcoming the former problem of obscuring the calibration markers with contrast. However, some fluoroscopy systems 'crop' the acquired measurement image such that the proximally placed calibration markers are deleted, so the precaution with this sizing balloon is to acquire a wider than usual field of interest. The third type of sizing balloon is a more spherical balloon which is advanced into the left atrium and inflated with a known injectate volume and withdrawn across the septum until it is just felt to pull through the septum. This is deemed a more subjective maneuver and is less favored because of the potential problem of enlarging the defect by tearing.

In the case of the AGA and PTS sizing balloon catheters, the balloon is advanced along the wire, crossing the atrial septum, and inflated gradually until the balloon is constrained by the edges of the defect. Overzealous inflation will obviously oversize the defect. A left anterior oblique projection of 30–45° with or without cranial angulation is commonly used. Using the calibration markers, the defect diameter is measured and the appropriate device size chosen. Some operators size smaller defects with well developed margins without the use of a balloon, relying exclusively on the TEE or intracardiac echo measurements.

The balloon and wire assembly are removed from the short sheath and the appropriate-sized HELEX device is flushed and withdrawn into its delivery catheter where more flushing is recommended until the system is completely de-aired. The loaded delivery catheter is advanced under fluoroscopic control to the right atrium, thence to the mid-cavity of the left atrium. Under fluoroscopic guidance the left atrial disk of the device is configured using a series of pushing and pulling maneuvers with alternate pushing of the control catheter and pulling of the mandrel. Complete configuration of the left disk is seen when the central eyelet of the device is at the end of the delivery catheter. The delivery system is then pulled to the atrial septum and alignment of the left disk against the septum confirmed on transesophageal echocardiography. The right atrial aspect of the device is configured using a pushing maneuver of the control catheter with the mandrel locked in a static position. At this stage both disks are seen clearly on echocardiography and any residual shunt is evident. Understandably a small amount of residual shunting through the device (as opposed to around the edges) is common at this stage. If the device configuration appears satisfactory it is then locked by first removing the red safety cap and then pulling firmly on the mandrel with the delivery system kept immobile (Figure 9.3a–c). The position of the device is assessed echocardiographically; if the device appears stable within the ASD, the delivery catheter is removed slowly under fluoroscopic control until the full length of the suture has run through the proximal eyelet and the device is fully free of the delivery catheter. If for any reason the device position is suboptimal, it is possible to make small adjustments to its position and constitution by first replacing the red safety cap and sliding the delivery catheter along the suture to the proximal eyelet. Small movements of the delivery catheter can then be made to alter the position of the device whilst observing under TEE guidance.[6] Once this has been achieved the red cap is removed and the delivery system withdrawn as described above. If, after locking, the device position is unacceptable and cannot be adjusted satisfactorily, the HELEX device can be removed in its entirety by replacing the red safety cap and pulling the device firmly into the delivery catheter and thus out of the patient. The procedure is covered by a single dose of heparin (100 U/kg) and with procedure times usually less than one hour, it is not usual practice to monitor activated clotting time (ACT). If for any reason the procedure is prolonged, then further doses of heparin to keep the ACT in the region of 200–250 s are recommended. Prophylactic antibiotics are given with induction of anesthesia and are usually institution specific. Most patients stay overnight in hospital undergoing an ECG and echocardiogram the morning following the procedure, but some centers regularly perform ASD closure as a day case

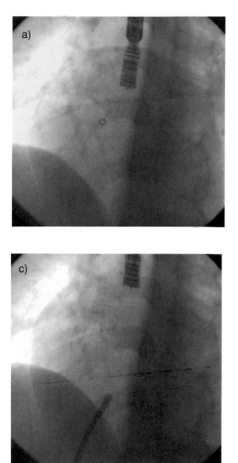
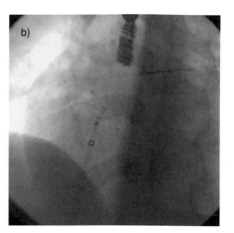

Figure 9.3 Stepwise fluoroscopic images of HELEX device deployment. a) Left atrial disk configured and pulled to septum. b) Both disks constituted either side of atrial septum. c) Post release, device detached completely from delivery system.

procedure with an echocardiogram some four hours or so afterwards prior to discharge. An antiplatelet dose of aspirin given once daily for six months is virtually universal practice. Some centers add a two month course of clopidogrel for adult patients. Follow-up at six weeks, six months and one year is common practice with ECG and echocardiographic assessment on each occasion. It is my practice to follow children until they have finished growing, but this is not universal practice.

PATENT FORAMEN OVALE CLOSURE

The HELEX device with its characteristics of flexibility, low profile, and low thrombogenicity make it an eminently suitable device with which to close the patent foramen ovale in patients with cryptogenic stroke. The device is suited to all types of PFO except perhaps those associated with a long flap-like tunnel in excess of 8 mm from the right atrial to left atrial aspect. Closure rates approach 100% actuarily, thrombus formation and recurrence of cerebrovascular events are very low.[7-9] The device delivery procedure is virtually identical save for the use of the monorail technique. This is helpful practically when it is acknowledged that on occasions it can be difficult to cross a PFO even with a diagnostic catheter. In this circumstance the femoral vein sheath should be 12Fr gauge. The PFO is crossed with the diagnostic catheter to the left atrium and into the left upper pulmonary vein, and a heavy duty type guide-wire positioned. The HELEX device is loaded into the delivery catheter in the normal way and withdrawn 2 cm proximal to the tip. The guide-wire is then introduced through the monorail port close to the tip of the delivery catheter and run through the sheath and forward to the left atrium. The guide-wire is then withdrawn and the device constituted as described above. Follow-up is much the same as for ASD with perhaps more centers opting for the addition of clopidogrel to aspirin therapy. Most patients undergoing PFO closure are already pretreated with aspirin.

In order to avoid the need for general anesthesia for simultaneous cardiac catheterization and transesophageal echocardiography, intracardiac echocardiography is gaining in popularity for PFO closure. This technique gives high-quality images of all parts of the atrial septum facilitating sizing and closure technique (Figure 9.4).

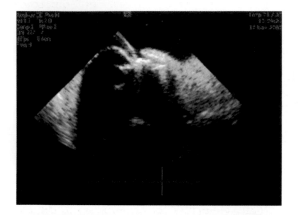

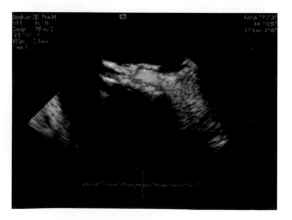

Figure 9.4 Intracardiac echocardiographic images of PFO closure. a) Left atrial disk pulled to the atrial septum. b) Appearance of HELEX device post release. Flexible molding of the device to the atrial septum is apparent.

CLOSURE OF FENESTRATED FONTAN

The term 'Fontan' circulation has come to encompass a variety of physiologic states which have in common the surgical connection of systemic veins to the pulmonary arteries. This is a form of radical palliation constituted to alleviate symptoms and prolong life in patients who essentially have only one functional ventricle. The most frequent intracardiac substrate is that of tricuspid atresia, but this palliation is also applied to patients with a hypoplastic left ventricle and a whole range of single ventricle physiologic states. In its commonest form, the superior vena cava is anastomosed to the right pulmonary artery and, at a later date, inferior vena caval blood is directed to the main pulmonary artery. This latter maneuver is usually accomplished using either a hemicylinder of prosthetic material (usually Goretex or Dacron) within the right atrium, so-called creation of a 'lateral tunnel'. Alternatively, and increasingly commonly, inferior vena cava bloodflow is connected to the main pulmonary artery using a tube of prosthetic material placed as an extracardiac conduit directing hepatic and inferior caval blood to the pulmonary artery. Surgical selection for this form of palliation is dependent on many variables of anatomy and physiology, some of which can often only be partly objective. As a precaution it is often desirable to create a 'fenestration' in the lateral tunnel or extracardiac conduit to act as a pressure-relieving 'blow off valve'. This usually takes the form of a 4 or 5 mm coronary punch hole. This enables right-to-left shunting of blood into the left atrial side of the circulation; though this results in desaturation of the patient, cardiac output is maintained should the hemodynamics be otherwise suboptimal. In most cases such fenestrations close spontaneously in the weeks and months following surgery, but occasionally it is necessary for reasons of desaturation to close them interventionally to improve oxygenation and avoid the risk of systemic thromboembolism. The small 15 mm HELEX device is ideal for such fenestrations because of its low profile, flexibility, and low thrombogenicity in a circulation which is acknowledged to be at risk of venous stagnation and thromboembolic complication.[10]

In most instances, venous access is from the femoral vein, but occasionally, because of congenital or acquired problems of inferior vena caval drainage, an internal jugular or even transhepatic venous approach is necessary. A diagnostic catheter is advanced from the femoral vein across the fenestration to the left atrium and, with the aid of a wire, into one of the pulmonary veins. The HELEX device is loaded normally and the delivery catheter advanced using the monorail port as described above. The technique of constituting the left and right atrial disks of the device is identical to that described for ASD and PFO closure. Figure 9.5 demonstrates closure of a fenestrated Fontan in a patient with a lateral tunnel cavopulmonary connection.

Many institutions as a matter of course administer warfarin anticoagulation to patients with a Fontan type circulation; this may be instead of or in addition to low-dose aspirin. Such patients are scrutinized regularly in any case for signs of thrombi in the lateral tunnel/extracardiac conduit.

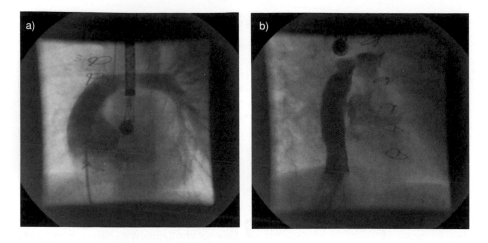

Figure 9.5   HELEX device closure of a fenestrated lateral tunnel cavopulmonary connection. a) Angiogram showing right-to-left shunting through fenestration in lateral tunnel. b) Angiogram immediately following implantation of a 15 mm HELEX device showing trivial residual shunting.

PROBLEMS, RISKS, COMPLICATIONS

Implantation of intracardiac devices for many adult-based cardiologists is a very different procedure to that of coronary stent implantation, where much of their interventional skills will lie. Whilst many cardiologists will perform hundreds of angioplasty procedures in a year, even the busiest, with an adult congenital bias or referral base, will in the European context close fewer than 50 ASDs and PFOs in a year. Factoring in the expertise of becoming familiar with the technical operation of the device, and its appearance and performance fluoroscopically, on transesophageal echocardiography, and subsequently intracardiac echocardiography, it should be recognized that a period of a 'learning curve' with close proctoring by an experienced operator is desirable.[11,12] The HELEX device has its positive attributes in its appeal as proven biocompatible material in the circulation, but there are several stages to its loading, deployment and release, and to its recovery should there be an unsatisfactory configuration or embolization. Those wishing to use the HELEX device are well advised to seek peer proctoring until they are comfortable with case selection, technical knowledge of the device, and familiarity and confidence in dealing with straightforward and more complex cases.

Retrieval of a device which has deployed unsatisfactorily with premature locking or displacement can be performed using the safety retrieval suture secured in position with the red safety cap. For device embolization after complete deployment you are recommended to position a 10 or 11Fr long sheath in the proximity of the embolized device and to use a 'goose neck' or other snare catheter to retrieve it into the sheath and thus out of the circulation. Remember that most cases of embolization are as a result of inadvertent undersizing of the defect and implantation of a larger device should be considered to complete therapy (Figure 9.6).

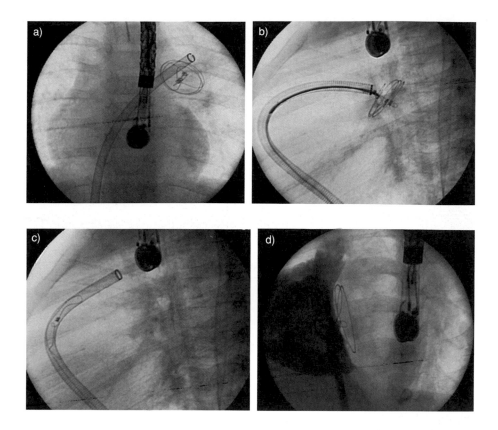

Figure 9.6 Retrieval of a 20 mm HELEX device which had embolized to the left pulmonary artery using a goose neck snare through a long 10Fr sheath. In this patient a 25 mm device was deployed after retrieval achieving closure of the ASD. a) 20 mm HELEX device embolized to left pulmonary artery. b) Device secured with goose neck snare via long 10Fr sheath. c) Device removed via long 10Fr sheath. d) Right atrial angiogram following closure with a 25 mm device.

CONCLUSIONS

Cardiologists are fortunate now in having a range of devices with which to close intracardiac defects. Accepting comparable safety and efficacy, biocompatibility and ease of use issues become imporant in the selection of devices for the catheter lab. Audit and clinical governance would direct us that achieving expertise in a number of different devices is logical, though rules of avoiding 'occasional practice' would dictate that all cardiologists could not use all devices. We should also keep an eye to the future, assessing how devices may perform in the growing heart. Likewise, technical and material advances will evolve and we should be prepared to embrace them.

REFERENCES

1. Zahn EM, Wilson N, Cutright W, Latson LA. Development and testing of the HELEX septal occluder, a new expanded polytetrafluoroethylene atrial septal defect occlusion system. Circulation 2001; 104:711–6.
2. Latson LA, Zahn EM, Wilson N. HELEX septal occluder for closure of atrial septal defects. Curr Interv Cardiol Rep 2000; 3:268–73.
3. Dobrolet NC, Iskowitz S, Lopez L, Whalen R, Zahn EM. Sequential implantation of two HELEX septal occluder devices in a patient with complex atrial septal anatomy. Catheter Cardiovasc Interv 2001; 2:242–6.
4. Pedra CA, Pedra SR, Esteves CA et al. Transcatheter closure of secundum atrial septal defects with complex anatomy. J Invasive Cardiol 2004; 16(3):117–22.
5. Krumsdorf U, Keppeler P, Horvath K, Zadan E, Schrader R, Sievert H. Catheter closure of atrial septal defects and patent foramen ovale in patients with an atrial septal aneurysm using different devices. J Interv Cardiol 2001; 1:49–55.
6. Lopez L, Ventura R, Welch EM, Nykanen DG, Zahn EM. Echocardiographic considerations during deployment of the HELEX septal occluder for closure of atrial septal defects. Cardiol Young 2003; 3:290–8.
7. Sievert H, Horvath K, Zadan E et al. Patent foramen ovale closure in patients with transient ischemia attack/stroke. J Interv Cardiol 2001; 2:261–6.
8. Onorato E, Melzi G, Casilli F et al. Patent foramen ovale with paradoxical embolism: mid-term results of catheter closure in 256 patients. J Interv Cardiol 2003; 1:43–50.
9. Krumsdorf U, Ostermayer S, Billinger K et al. Incidence and clinical course of thrombus formation on atrial septal defect and patent foramen ovale closure devices in 1000 consecutive patients. J Am Coll Cardiol 2004; 2:302–9.
10. Peuster M, Beerbaum P. A novel implantation technique for closure of an atypical fenestration connecting the right atrial appendage to an extracardiac conduit by use of a 15mm HELEX device in a patient with a total cavopulmonary connection. Z Kardiol 2004; 10:818–23.
11. Vincent RN, Raviele AA, Diehl HJ. Single center experience with the HELEX septal occluder for closure of atrial septal defects in children. J Interv Cardiol 2003; 1:79–82.
12. Pedra CA, Pedra SF, Esteves CA et al. Initial experience in Brazil with the HELEX septal occluder for percutaneous occlusion of atrial septal defects. Arq Bras Cardiol 2003; 5:435–52.

10

Closure of interatrial communications using the CardioSEAL/STARFlex devices

Igor F Palacios

Introduction • Atrial septal defects • Ventricular septal defects • Patent foramen ovale • Surgical treatment • Transcatheter management • The NMT family of septal occluders • Implantation technique • Clinical results

INTRODUCTION

In this chapter, I will attempt to provide a brief overview, and address trans-catheter management of common interatrial communications using the CardioSEAL®/STARFlex® occluder devices. We will consider three major types of atrial septal defects: secundum, primum, and sinus venosus, and the PFO.

ATRIAL SEPTAL DEFECTS

Atrial septal defects (ASDs) represent an abnormality in the development of the heart that results in free communication between the atria compared to patent foramen ovale, which represents the persistence of normal fetal cardiovascular physiology. ASDs are categorized according to their anatomy as follows.

Ostium secundum atrial septal defects are considered to be the third most common form of congenital heart disorder; they represent 80% of all ASDs and are one of the most common congenital cardiac malformations in adults, accounting for 30% to 40% of these patients over the age of 40. Ostium secundum describes defects that are located midseptally and are typically near the fossa ovalis.

Ostium primum defects lie immediately adjacent to the atrioventricular valves and occur commonly in patients with Down's syndrome.

Sinus venous defects occur high in the atrial *septum* and are frequently associated with anomalies of the pulmonary veins.

The defect often goes unnoticed for decades because the physical signs are subtle and the clinical symptoms are mild. The majority of patients have few symptoms; fatigue and shortness of breath are the most common complaints. However, virtually all patients who survive into their sixth decade are sympto-matic; less than 50% of patients survive beyond 40 to 50 years due to heart failure or pulmonary hypertension related to the left-to-right shunt. Patients with ASDs are also at risk for paradoxical emboli. Therefore, repair of ASDs is recommended for those patients with pulmonary to systemic flows exceeding 1.5:1.0. Because most have no symptoms, atrial septal defects most often are discovered on pre-school entrance examinations when the physician hears a murmur and investigates it. The diagnosis is confirmed by echocardiography, which may visualize the actual defect and estimate its size, as well as the connection of the pulmonary veins. Cardiac catheterization is indicated in cases of an inconclusive echocardiographic examination or associated anomalies which require further evaluation or as part of patients undergoing catheter closure of the ASD. Twenty per cent of atrial septal defects will close spontaneously in the first year of life. One percent becomes symptomatic in the first year, with an associated 0.1% mortality. There is a 25% lifetime risk of mortality in unrepaired atrial septal defects. The risk factors associated with increased mortality include the development of pulmonary vascular obstructive disease. This is why we electively close ASDs which have not closed spontaneously by school-age.

Certain types of ASDs (sinus venosus and primum varieties) have no chance of spontaneous closure, and patients with these types are not candidates for transcatheter closure because of the location of the ASD. Open-heart surgery is indicated for patients with these types of ASDs.

Despite the success of operative repair, there has been interest in developing a catheter-based approach to ASD repair in order to avoid the risks and morbidity of open-heart surgery. Recent developments have enabled cardiologists to close congenital defects, such as a patent ductus arteriosus, a ventricular septal defect, and atrial septal defects. Interventional cardiologists can close these defects during cardiac catheterization, avoiding the need for general anesthesia, thoracotomy, and extended stays in the hospital; thus, significantly reducing medical costs.

A variety of devices have been researched over the past 20 years; technical challenges include minimizing the size of the device so that smaller catheters can be used; developing techniques to properly center the device across the ASD, and ensuring that the device can be easily retrieved or repositioned if necessary. Late failures due to mechanical stress have also been a concern. Early devices such as the Rashkind hook device and the Lock Clamshell device were limited by their large size and technical malfunctions.

Current devices under investigation include the Sideris buttoned device, the Das Angel Wings device, the Atrial Septal Defect Occluding System (ASDOS), the HELEX device, and the CardioSEAL® and STARFlex® devices (Figure 10.1). At the present time, the Amplatzer® Septal Occluder (by AGA Medical Corp) is the only septal occlusion device to have been FDA-approved for the occlusion of atrial septal defects in secundum position. While most devices attempt to patch the ASD, the Amplatzer® device is unique in that it consists in part of an atherogenic stent designed to promote thrombosis of the ASD. The CardioSEAL® device, which has been FDA-approved for the treatment of PFO, is also under investigation for atrial septal defects and has been used for ASD as an off-label indication. The STARFlex® device is undergoing evaluation in patients with PFO and cryptogenic stroke (CLOSURE I trial) and in patients with PFO and migraine with aura (MIST trials I and II).

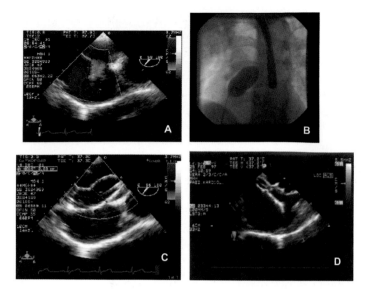

Figure 10.1   Catheter closure of secundum ASD using the CardioSEAL®/STARFlex® occluder device. Panel A: TEE of a patient undergoing catheter closure of a secundum ASD. Panel B: Stretched balloon sizing of ASD diameter. A waist produced by the defect is seen in the sizing balloon catheter. This waist is associated with no evidence of shunting as assessed by TEE. Panel C: Echocardiographic measurement of stretched balloon diameter of the secundum ASD. Panel D: Optimal deployment of 40 mm CardioSEAL® device to occlude the secundum ASD.

VENTRICULAR SEPTAL DEFECTS

Ventricular septal defect (VSD) is an abnormal opening in the septum that separates the right and left ventricles. It is the most common congenital defect of the heart. It is estimated that up to 0.4% of babies are born with this condition. The hole is small in a vast majority of the babies; they will have no symptoms as the defect will spontaneously close as the muscular wall continues to grow. If the communication is large, too much blood will be pumped into the lungs, leading to congestive heart failure. CardioSEAL® Septal Occlusion System with QuickLoad™ was FDA-approved in December 2001 for use in closing ventricular septal defects.

PATENT FORAMEN OVALE

The foramen ovale is an opening between the right and left atrium that functions as a vascular bypass of the uninflated lungs of a fetus prior to birth. Within several months following birth, the opening normally closes permanently as the result of increased left atrial pressure and decreased right atrial pressure. Although usually clinically insignificant, patent foramen ovales are found in approximately 10–25% of adult patients. In these patients, the PFO is more often associated with paradoxical embolus where an embolus in the venous circulation gains access to the arterial circulation, resulting in a stroke or transient ischemic attack (TIA). PFOs are typically closed by open surgery or transcatheter approaches. Treatment alternatives include chronic anticoagulation therapy, based in part on the theory that clotting disorders may be present in patients with embolic stroke. The CardioSEAL® Septal Occlusion System was FDA-approved through a Humanitarian Device Exemption (HDE) in February 2000 for the treatment of patent foramen ovale. The Amplatzer® PFO Occluder was FDA-approved under this same exemption program in April 2002 for use in the closure of a PFO.

SURGICAL TREATMENT

Indications for surgical repair of an atrial septal defect are right ventricular over-load (due to flow from the left atrium into the right atrium), a shunt fraction with a pulmonary to systemic flow ratio > 2.0 as estimated by echocardiography, and elective closure prior to a child starting school. The surgical treatment options for an ASD closure include direct suture repair, which is reserved for small atrial septal defects, and the more common patch repair. The material utilized for patch closure of ASDs may be the patient's own pericardium, commercially available bovine pericardium, or synthetic material (Gore-Tex, Dacron). The surgical approach to the atrial septal defect is somewhat dependent upon its location and could be performed by median sternotomy, right thoracotomy, and submammary approach.

All types of ASDs may be approached adequately through a median ster-notomy or right thoracotomy. The submammary incision may be the most cosmetic, but makes some ASDs difficult to repair. The primary benefits of the submammary and thoracotomy incisions are cosmetic in nature. The term 'mini-mally invasive surgery' for repair of atrial septal defects usually refers to repair of the defect using the same techniques as open-heart surgical repair that is, using cardiopulmonary bypass, but performing the operation through a much smaller incision. Most children can successfully undergo this type of repair through a small (3–4 inches) incision in the sternum. In general, the postopera-tive course in the hospital is shorter (2–3 days), due to less incisional pain and discomfort. Once the pericardium is opened, regardless of the choice of inci-sions, the patient is placed on cardiopulmonary bypass and blood is diverted away from the right atrium. High-potassium cardioplegia is then administered after the aorta is clamped, thus stopping the heart. The right atrium is then opened to allow access to the atrial septum below. Dependent upon the size and location of the defect, it may be closed directly with sutures or with a patch. Once the defect is closed, the atrial incision is closed as well. The aortic cross clamp is removed, and after normal ventilation is resumed, the patient is warmed and a stable rhythm is achieved, the patient may be weaned from cardiopulmonary bypass. A single drainage tube is placed and the chest is closed. The results of surgical repair of atrial septal defects are excellent. Surgical mortality is less than one percent, and average hospital stay is four days. These results indicate that ASDs of all types may be effectively repaired in infants and children with very low mortality and morbidity. Optimal timing for surgery in the asymptomatic child remains prior to starting grade school. The asympto-matic child with an atrial septal defect deserves close follow-up by the pediatri-cian and pediatric cardiologist, with constant involvement of the cardiovascular surgeon. Should a patient become symptomatic with failure to thrive, or persistent complaints (malaise, respiratory infections, etc.), early surgical intervention would be warranted.

TRANSCATHETER MANAGEMENT

To date, the primary method of therapy for closure of the atrial septal defect has been surgical repair. As with all forms of cardiac surgery, there is a small but definite risk of surgical morbidity (5%) and mortality (<1%). Reports of very early results (1950s to 1960s) revealed fairly high death rates and complication rates. In the 1990s, however, marked improvement in surgical technique has contributed to the significantly improved outcomes reported above.

In light of this history, interventional cardiologists explored the possibility of transcatheter closure of the atrial septal defect. This technique involves implantation of one of several devices (basically single or double wire frames covered by fabric) using heart catheterization methods in the cardiac catheterization laboratory, without the need for cardiopulmonary bypass, and without the need to stop the heart.[1–8] The ideal closure device is not available. The ideal delivery system/closure device should be user-friendly and be able to be retrieved or repositioned. It should achieve an effective/high complete closure rate and be advanced through a small introducer. It should have a self-centering mechanism. It should have durability until full endothelialization, and must preserve flow and function despite embolization. Finally it must be economical, and competitive with surgical closure.

The appropriate selection of patients for this technology is rather strict, and is mainly limited by the Food and Drug Administration guidelines. Obvious evidence of enlargement of the right heart by chest X-ray, cardiac ultrasound, or previous angiography, or recurrent and frequent lung infections would be principal indicators for closure of these defects. Defects amenable to such device therapy tend to be smaller (less than 20 to 25 mm in diameter). Importantly, these lesions must be centrally located within the atrial septum. Defects at the very upper or lower edges of the atrial septum (called ostium primum or sinus venosus) are not good candidates for this procedure, because these defects usually involve other abnormalities of the heart valves, or venous drainage from the lungs.

Recent data suggest that patients with these types of defects, and a prior history of stroke, may be at a higher risk of stroke recurrence without closure of the atrial defect. At present there are no lower age limitations, which preclude device implantation. In many cases, because of the size of the device and its introduction system device, applicability may be limited to patients who weigh more than 8 to 10 kg (18 to 22 lb).

The usual procedure is very similar to standard heart catheterization. Briefly, flexible catheters are inserted into the veins and arteries in the groin. The patient should undergo routine right and left heart catheterization with measurement of pressures and oxygen levels in all of the chambers of the heart. Angiograms are performed to determine the size of the chambers, the size of the defect, and its location within the heart. Using a balloon catheter of a known diameter, the defect is then sized in comparison to the balloon, so that the device appropriate for that particular patient can be chosen. The device is then advanced into the heart through a Mullins sheath introducer. With most of the presently used devices, half of the device is connected to one side of the atrial septum, and the second half of the device attached to the other portion, forming a sort of 'sandwich' of the defect. Within six to eight weeks, the device acts as a 'skeleton' or a 'framework', which stimulates normal tissue to grow in and over the defect. This is how, for example, these devices can be used in growing children; though the device itself does not grow, the tissue that covers the device does, and will continue to grow as the child grows. The time and degree of tissue coverage is still under investigation. The entire procedure is performed under general or local anesthesia, and the actual implantation of the device is performed using either transesophageal or intracardiac echocardiographic guidance respectively (Figure 10.1).

As described above, there are multiple devices presently being tested under FDA guidelines. In general, successful closure of these defects using a device occurs in 80–95% of patients with no significant leak through the defects (Tables 10.1–10.3).

The major advantage of this technology is its relative non-invasive approach. Patients are usually hospitalized overnight, and many return to work or school

Table 10.1   Residual shunt post interatrial communication closure

Device	Pts	24 h	6 months	1 year	3 years	5 years
Sideris IV (1)	423	38%	32%	29%	12%	0%
Amplatzer® (2)	1931	19%	6%	5%	–	–
CardioSEAL® (3–4)	132	11%	6%	–	–	–
Angel Wings (5)	70	18%	8%	–	–	–

(1) North American Multicenter Trial, AHA 1999.
(2) Amplatzer® Registry, 1999.
(3) North American Multicenter Trial, AHA 1998.
(4) European Multicenter Trial, AHA 1998.
(5) Banerjee A et al. Am J Cardiol 1999; 83:1236–1241.

Table 10.2   Immediate and 1-year follow-up effective occlusion after interatrial communication closure

Device	Pts	Immediate	1 Year F/U
Sideris IV (1)	242	86%	93%
Amplatzer® (2)	1931	97%	100%
CardioSEAL® (3–4)	132	89%	94%
Angel Wings (5)	88	–	95%

(1) North American Multicenter Trial, AHA 1999.
(2) Amplatzer® Registry, 1999.
(3) North American Multicenter Trial, AHA 1998.
(4) European Multicenter Trial, AHA 1998.
(5) Banerjee A et al. Am J Cardiol 1999; 83:1236–1241.

Table 10.3 Immediate and long-term outcomes of interatrial communications closure

Author	Patients	Age	Successful deployment	Immediate closure rate	Death	Surgery	Stroke	Recurrent neuro events	1-year residual shunt
Varma Ch	92	45±13	100%	95%	0%	0%	0%	2.7%	10%
Brown PG	100		100%	75%	0%	0%	0%		
Somers RJ	265	50	100%	88%	0%	0%	2%	1.4%	1.9%
Bialkowski	209	20	96%	100%	0%	0%	0%		0.0%
Carminati M	117	17	100%		0%	0%	0%	20.5%	
Buttera	121	20±17	100%						
Knebel F	161	47±11	100%						
Hammon H	100	52	100%						
Rao	423		90%		1.4%			14%	
Tuzcu V	129		92%					2%	2%
Martin F	110		100%	100%	0%	0%	0%	0.9%	0%
Block PC	100		100%	71%	0%	0%	0%		

within 1–2 days. We have had patients who have been able to resume vigorous exercise (horseback riding and competitive sports) within weeks or months after device implantation. Compiling data for all the presently tested devices, the complication rate following transcatheter ASD occlusion is approximately 5%. These complications include the routine risks of cardiac catheterization such as vascular injury, particularly in cases where larger device introducer systems need to be used. Sometimes, problems with blood clotting or excessive bleeding may be seen, particularly in younger patients.

A rare complication unique to this technology may be the possibility of clot formation on the device itself,[3,9] with the risk of breakage of the clot causing stroke, or a clot into the vessels of the lung (pulmonary embolus). At present, these problems are addressed by using adequate doses of aspirin or warfarin following the procedure, and by using heparin during the procedure to reduce the clotting factors within the blood. The aspirin or warfarin is used for three to six months, until we are sure that the device is fully scarred in place, and incorporated into the atrial tissue.

The length of and need for antibiotic bacterial endocarditis prophylaxis vary amongst investigators and devices, lasting from 12 months following device implant to life-long administration. Most patients are followed at 1, 3, and 6 months, and then, for 1, 2, 3, 4, and 5 years after device implantation with variable requirements for echocardiograms, chest X-rays and electrocardiograms. Residual shunt is determined by 2-D echocardiography, color flow Doppler, and agitated saline solution contrast injection into an antecubital vein and categorized as follows: 0, none, indicating no microbubbles in the left atrium after administration of agitated saline; 1, small, indicating the presence of 3 to 9 microbubbles in the left atrium after the administration of agitated saline; 2, moderate, indicating 10 to 30 microbubbles in the left atrium after administration of agitated saline; and 3, large, >30 microbubbles in the left atrium after administration of agitated saline. For purposes of analysis and data comparison of immediate and long-term results, 'effective occlusion' refers to the combination of none or small shunt post device implantation. Figure 10.2 shows changes in residual shunt after CardioSEAL® implantation as assessed by the former echocardiographic classification of patients who underwent catheter closure of interatrial communications (PFO or small ASD) using the CardioSEAL® occluder device. As shown in Figure 10.2, an effective occlusion was achieved in all patients immediately after device implantation. During the follow-up period there was a progressive increase in the number of patients achieving total occlusion that reached 100% by one year of follow-up.

Certainly this technology is not for everyone. However, if patients are properly selected, the results of device closure of the atrial septal defect may prove to be, in many cases, equivalent to those results obtained through standard surgical intervention without some of the issues involved with open heart surgery.

Atrial septal defects are treated successfully using transcatheter techniques. In 1975, King et al. were the first ones to attempt a transcatheter closure of an atrial septal defect. They used a double-umbrella system, which was placed across the atrial septal defect via a large delivery catheter to close the atrial communication. A single umbrella-type device was then developed (Rashkind), consisting of polyurethane foam, mounted on a stainless steel skeleton with six arms radiating out of the hub. Every other arm had a small barbed hook at a

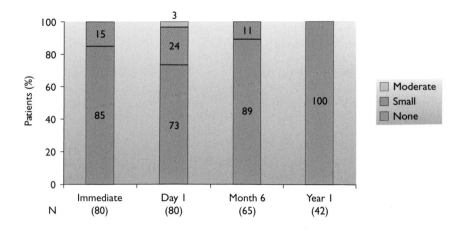

Figure 10.2 Changes in residual shunt after CardioSEAL® device implantation as assessed by echocardiography.

right angle to the arm. This single disk system is then folded up into a 15.5 French delivery system and delivered through a 16F sheath. Major limitations of this device were: (1) its size; (2) the location of the defect that could be closed; and (3) the use of a hook device that did not allow the system to be retrieved if improperly positioned. A greater improvement in the closure of atrial septal defects occurred during the last years. Several devices underwent and are undergoing clinical trials in the United States including the Clamshell Septal Occluder device, the Siderid buttoned device, the Das self-centering double disk device and more recently the Amplatz self-centering device (see Tables 10.1–10.3). Table 10.3 depicts immediate and long-term results of different occluder devices used to close percutaneously ASD and PFO.[4–33]

Large clinical trials have been performed with the Clamshell and the Buttoned device. The results were good in both methods with a low morbidity and mortality in selected patients with atrial septal defect. James Lock introduced the double-hinged 'clamshell' umbrella occluding device in 1989. This device allowed the arms to fold back again using a spring tension, rather than a hook, to fit the device on the atrial septum. The clamshell configuration of the distal arms could be diverted during device placement, thus, creating a cone that would self-center and allow easy device repositioning. The size of the delivery pod was reduced to 11 French, and the foam modified, so as to make a more occlusive device. With this device, atrial septal defects up to 2 cm in diameter in the secundum position can be successfully closed using transcatheter closure techniques. It is necessary to measure the size of the atrial septal defect. This can be accomplished non-invasively by using two-dimensional echocardiography, transesophageal echocardiography, and nuclear magnetic resonance. Cardiac angiography and direct sizing of the atrial septal defect using balloon sizing catheters are used at the time of cardiac catheterization (Figure 10.1). However, arm fractures occurred often after the implantation of the Clamshell device. The frequency was 75% and 43% for ASD and PFO closures respectively.

The buttoned Sideris device is a double disk device consisting of a square-shaped polyurethane folding disk with two stainless steel skeleton wires, called an occluder, a rhomboid-shaped, single wire polyurethane disk with a latex valve sutured at its center, called a counteroccluder, and a nylon loop sutured at the center of the occluder. The Sideris device has been implanted in more than 1,000 patients and some of these are documented in United States, European, and international trial reports. The long-term success rate of an implanted device should range between 95% and 98% for a wide range of secundum atrial septal defects with favorable anatomy. Clinical trials were carried out with the Das 'angel wings' device in 75 patients with secundum ASD with a diameter ≤ 20 mm. The device was successfully deployed in 72 (96%) patients. A residual shunt was present in 27% of the patients immediately after the procedure, transient complete AV block occurred in three (4%) patients and the right atrial disk was not fully deployed in three patients. A minor shunt (< 3 mm in diameter) was present only in three (4%) of 72 patients during follow-up of 1–17 months. Blood clots in the right atrial disk were present in two patients. Serious complications demanding surgical removal of the device occurred in three patients. One patient had hemopericardium and tamponade because of an aortic lesion, another patient had left atrial thrombus formation due to an unfolded right atrial disk, and the last patient had dislodgment of the left atrial disk and a large residual shunt. Thus, it appears that the device should be modified as 4% of the patients had serious complications.[11]

Potential candidates for transcatheter closure of atrial septal defects are those patients with communications located in the secundum position measuring ≤ 20 mm in their largest diameter. Inclusion criteria include echocardiographic features of ostium secundum ASD; with QP:QS > 1.5:1; with adequate rim of atrial septum surrounding the ASD (≤ 4 mm away from important structures, i.e. coronary sinus, AV valves and pulmonary veins. A deficient anterior ring is not a contraindication as the posterior wall of the aortic root provides anterior support to the device); stretched ASD diameter ≤ 20 mm for the no self-center devices, and ≤ 34 mm for the self-center ASD Amplatzer®; or PFO causing paradoxical embolism, or platypnea/orthodeoxia and hypoxemia, and/or cyanosis due to right-to-left shunting.

All patients should undergo standard right and left heart catheterization, left atrial cine angiography and measurement of the defect using sizing balloons, which have been passed through the atrial communication. If the defect is judged to be in good position, to have an appropriate size and adequate margins, an 11 French Mullins' sheath is passed from the femoral vein, into the left atrium and the left upper pulmonary vein. The patients are premedicated using a standard medication for cardiac catheterization. General anesthesia and transesophageal echocardiography are used as a routine by some investigators while other interventionists prefer conscious sedation, local anesthesia, and intracardiac echocardiography. Patients are fully heparinized and prophylactic intravenous antibiotics are used beginning two hours before the procedure. When using the clamshell device or any of the NMT family of occluder devices, the occluding device is advanced through the sheath until the delivery pod on the end of the catheters reaches the level of the tricuspid valve. At this point, the sheath is used as an extension of the pod. The delivery wire is advanced slowly, delivering the occluder out of the pod into the sheath. The delivery wire continues to be advanced until the occluder is at the end of the sheath. The entire delivery system, including the sheath and the catheter, can now be withdrawn into the left atrium. The delivery wire is then advanced carefully until the distal set of arms is extruded from the sheath and the distal arms spring open in the left atrium and pulled back to the left atrial side of the atrial septal defect. The entire delivery system (sheath, catheter, delivery wire and device) is slowly withdrawn with a slight tension of the delivery wire, so that the proximal arms will not open until the appropriate position of the distal arm is obtained. This can be identified by resistance to further withdrawal, transesophageal or intra-cardiac echocardiography and angiography. When the distal arms are in proper position, the central delivery wire is held in place and the sheath is then retracted, allowing the proximal arms to spring open in the right atrial side of the atrial septum. If all is well, the release mechanism in the central wire control clamp is engaged, allowing the central control wire to release the occluder. The delivery system is then withdrawn into the sheath and removed. A right atrial angiogram with levophase is performed to check the position of the device and the presence of residual shunting through the atrial septum.

Patients are kept overnight. There is no need for further heparinization. An over-penetrated chest X-ray is taken six hours following the procedure and prior to discharge, as well as follow-up two-dimensional echocardiography. Patients are given aspirin, 1 tablet p.o. q.d. for six months. There is no need for systemic anticoagulation. Healing appears complete with endothelialization, within a few weeks of implantation (Figure 10.3).

A clinical trial for transcatheter closure of atrial septal defects, using the Lock clamshell device, was initiated in 1989. During the first year, this procedure was attempted in 94 patients with a mean age of 14.5 (range 0.5–76.5) years and mean weight of 32.5 (range 6.1–90.5) kg. The mean size of the defect was 12.3 (range 2–25) mm. Sixty-eight patients had a secundum atrial septal defect, five patients

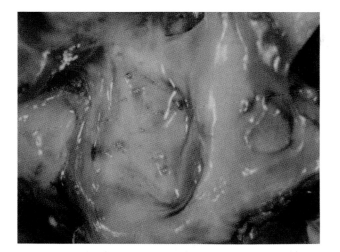

Figure 10.3   CardioSEAL® in a sheep heart explanted at 90 days.
Courtesy of Carol Devellian and Rudy Davis. NMT Medical, Boston, Massachusetts.

had patent foramen ovale and presented with paradoxical embolic strokes, 14 patients were status post fenestrated Fontan operation, and one patient had a residual atrial septal defect after percutaneous mitral balloon valvotomy. Placement of the device was achieved in 88 patients. Failure occurred in six patients; in three because of embolization due to sizing error, and in three because the defect was too big. Total closure has been achieved in more than 70% of the patients, a subtotal closure (indicates a leak around the device) was present in 22% of the cases. A failure (indicates that no device was left in place at the end of the case) was present in 6% of the cases. Complications were 5%. Complications encountered during this procedure have been related to embolization of the device from the atrial septum into either the pulmonary artery or the aorta. The system could be retrieved using retrieval catheters (basket, grabber, or forceps retrieval devices). At follow-up (1–6 months) there have been no embolizations, no strokes, no arrhythmias, and no subacute bacterial endocarditis.

The clamshell occluder device has also been used to close congenital and post myocardial infarction ventricular septal defects.

THE NMT FAMILY OF SEPTAL OCCLUDERS

The CardioSEAL®, STARFlex®, and BioStar® septal occluders (NMT Medical Inc., Boston, MA, USA) comprise three iterative generations of umbrella-type septal occluders, each designed to address evolving clinical demands as a result of expanded indications for use. NMT's occluder family is modeled after the original Clamshell™ device (C.R. Bard, Inc., Billerica, MA, USA), which remains the technological standard for devices. Umbrella-type septal occluders have been in clinical use since 1989 and are inherently appealing for closure of patent foramen ovale (PFO) due to (1) their excellent conformability to anatomic variations, maximizing closure rates while minimizing risk of erosion or perforation; (2) low septal profile to minimize hemodynamic disturbances; and (3) very low metal surface area to minimize risk of corrosive byproducts and maximize ability to recross the septum later in life. At the time of writing, the company estimates that over 20,000 patients in the US and Europe have been implanted for closure of PFO since 1996.

The CardioSEAL® septal occlusion system

The CardioSEAL®, shown in Figure 10.4, has the longest clinical use history of all currently available septal occluders. The double umbrella implant provides a highly conformable design with very low septal profile and low metal surface area. The implant consists of two identical umbrellas that sandwich the cardiac defect from both sides. Each umbrella consists of knitted polyester fabric supported by and fastened to four wire spring arms by polyester sutures. Each spring arm is constructed with a series of torsional springs strategically arranged and designed to control functional stresses in the wire and provide adequate fixation in the heart. The polyester tissue scaffold is well proven to promote endothelialization. The CardioSEAL® framework is fabricated from MP35n, a cobalt-based alloy known for its excellent corrosion resistance and MRI safety. As MP35n is not a shape memory material, it does not distort cardiac anatomy.

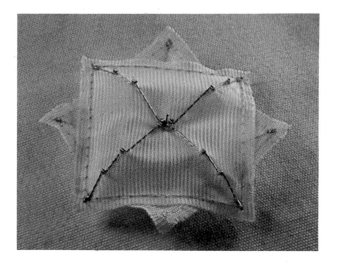

Figure 10.4   The CardioSEAL® occluder device. Courtesy of Carol Devellian and Rudy Davis. NMT Medical, Boston, Massachusetts.

The CardioSEAL® is available in four sizes: 17 mm, 23 mm, 28 mm, and 33 mm. Size is determined by the diagonal length of the metal arms. All four sizes are deliverable through an 11F sheath.

The CardioSEAL® received a CE Mark in Europe for closure of atrial level shunts in 1997. The CardioSEAL® is commercially available in the United States through an FDA Humanitarian Use Exemption (HDE) for the closure of a PFO in patients with recurrent cryptogenic stroke due to presumed paradoxical embolism through a PFO, and who have failed conventional drug therapy, and a Pre Market Approval (PMA) for closure of ventricular septal defects (VSDs) in high-risk patients.

The STARFlex® septal occlusion system

The STARFlex®, shown in Figures 10.5a and 10.5b, is similar to the CardioSEAL® in design and materials with the addition of an ultra-fine diameter wire (0.0015 inch) nitinol coil spring. The centering spring is continuous, with suture attachment points that alternate between the proximal and distal umbrellas. The centering spring is attached on the inside surface of each umbrella and therefore lies between the two pieces of fabric. Functionally, the centering spring positions the STARFlex® in the center of the PFO defect. This self-centering feature of the STARFlex® allows use of smaller-size devices relative to septal defect sizes while providing high rates of complete closure (97%[1]) and better apposition of the implant arms to the septal wall, important in closure of long tunnel PFOs. STARFlex® has a unique centering mechanism which auto-adjusts to center the STARFlex® within the PFO and assists in pulling the arms in tightly against the septal wall without distorting the septum, maximizing closure, and minimizing septal profile. The STARFlex® occluder is commercially available in Europe and is undergoing clinical trials for PFO – migraine and stroke indications – in both

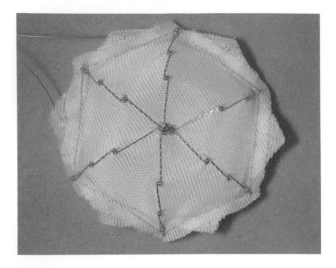

Figure 10.5a   The STARFlex® occluder device. Courtesy of Carol Devellian and Rudy Davis. NMT Medical, Boston, Massachusetts.

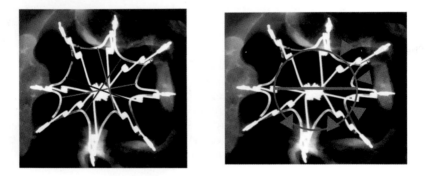

Figure 10.5b   Comparison of the STARFlex® vs. the Amplatzer® self-center devices. Digitally enhanced X-ray illustrating variations in lengths of ASD 'Radials'. With a STARFlex® occluder in place (right side panel) and same X-ray with a stent. Centering overlay illustrating areas where septum would be distorted by the stent (left side panel). Courtesy of Carol Devellian and Rudy Davis. NMT Medical, Boston, Massachusetts.

the US and Europe. These trials also incorporate the new Rapid Transport™ delivery system. Rapid Transport (or RT as it is called in the US) is a single-operator system with a pre-attached implant. This new system significantly simplifies the delivery process by reducing the number of steps to deliver an implant. It also allows accurate assessment of defect occlusion prior to implant release due to its unique attachment mechanism which allows for 180 degrees of rotation at the implant/delivery system interface. The STARFlex® occluder is available in four sizes: 23 mm, 28 mm, 33 mm, and 38 mm sizes. The 23 mm, 28 mm, and 33 mm devices have four arms per side while the 38 mm has six. The four-arm devices are deliverable through an 11F sheath, while the 38 mm requires a 12F.

Perceived disadvantages of the STARFlex® (and CardioSEAL®) septal occluders include retrieval complexity and lack of repositionability once fully deployed, and reports of device thrombosis.[2,3] The retrievability and repositioning concern is usually only an issue for the new user, but with proper training and sufficient experience, this concern is minimized. For PFO patients this is rarely, if ever, an issue. Nonetheless, when required, retrieval of a fully deployed device can be readily performed and is simplified by following a two-step procedure: first retrieving approximately half the umbrella into the long sheath, then retrieving the remaining umbrella into a previously back-loaded short sheath. It is important to use proper care to align the coils of the device within the sheath lumen when retracting the umbrella into the long sheath.

The risk of device thrombosis can be minimized through good patient screening, standardized procedural methodology, routine follow-up, and a standardized post implant drug regimen. The administration of protamine, used in some cases in the early years of PFO closure, is now recognized as a likely progenitor for thrombus in these patients, despite heparinization and administration of antiplatelet and/or anticoagulation agents peri-procedurally. In the modern implant era, defined as the time when the major randomized trials were initiated (2003), pharmacology has been standardized around aspirin and Plavix® both pre, and post implant, and the occasional addition of warfarin post implant for those patients who have coagulopathies, or other devices, that demand anticoagulation prophylaxis. Since that time, reports of thrombus have nearly disappeared.

The STARFlex® occluder received a CE Mark in Europe for closure of atrial level shunts in 1998. At writing, the STARFlex® is also being studied in four different clinical trials for closure of PFO (MIST, MIST II, MIST III, and CLOSURE I). In the United Kingdom, STARFlex® is being studied in a trial called MIST (Migraine Intervention with STARFlex® Technology) to evaluate the potential link between PFOs and migraine. At the time of writing, this trial was fully enrolled and followed-up and results were pending. In the United States, STARFlex® is being studied in two trials. The first, called CLOSURE I, is a 1,600 patient randomized, controlled clinical trial designed to evaluate the effectiveness of transcatheter PFO closure, compared to best medical therapy in stroke and TIA patients. The second US clinical trial is called MIST II and is similar in scope to the UK MIST trial described above.

The BioStar® septal occlusion system

The BioStar® is the first biological septal repair implant and continues the evolution of NMT septal occluders through the incorporation of a biologic material on the STARFlex® framework, representing the first bioabsorbable device in the septal occlusion space. The scaffold material is a tissue-engineered, highly purified acellular Type 1 collagen matrix derived from the submucosal layer of the porcine small intestine. Additionally, an ionically-bound heparin coating is added to decrease acute thrombogenicity while not adversely effecting the long-term healing response. The potential advantages of the BioStar® include more rapid defect sealing and endothelization, higher closure rates (both acute and long term), decreased thrombogenicity, improved chronic healing and closure of the intracardiac defect, and reduced obstruction access across the interatrial septum (in case left atrial access is required later in a patient's life). At writing, BioStar® is being studied clinically in the UK in the BEST (The BioStar® Evaluation Study) trial. It will be available in late 2006 in Europe in 23 mm, 28 mm, and 33 mm sizes deliverable by the Rapid Transport™ delivery system (RT in the US) and an 11F sheath.

Figure 10.6 depicts a BioStar® implanted in a freshly created defect. Note the nice adherence of the collagen matrix to the septal wall. The 30-day healing response of the BioStar® in the sheep model shows extensive tissue encapsulation and complete sealing to the atrial wall. Over time, the BioStar® collagen matrix remodels into native extracellular matrix.

IMPLANTATION TECHNIQUE

NMT is credited with the development and refinement of the technique for deployment of double umbrella type devices. Most procedures are done in the outpatient setting. The PFO closure technique will be described here.

All current implant devices incorporate the same basic technique. The procedure typically takes about 30 minutes in experienced hands, and requires only conscious sedation if intracardiac echo (ICE) is used. Echocardiographic and fluoroscopic guidance are requirements for effective placement and evaluation of outcome. The patient's vasculature is accessed most commonly via the right femoral vein, and the defect crossed with standard catheters and wires. Implant size determination may be done by either echo evaluation or by balloon assessment. Once determined, a Mullin's transseptal length sheath is placed across the defect, and the implant collapsed and transferred into the sheath. After advancing the implant to the defect, the distal umbrella is opened in the left

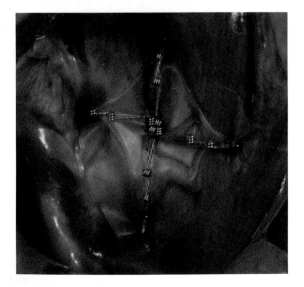

Figure 10.6 The BioSTAR® occluder device. Courtesy of Dr Christian Jux, University of Goettingen/Germany and Dr Peter Wohlsein, Institute of Pathology, School of Veterinary Medicine Hannover, Hannover/Germany.

atrium and the implant retracted back against the left atrial septal wall. At this point, if the implant position is satisfactory based on echocardiography and fluoroscopy, the right atrial umbrella is deployed, its position on the septum assessed again, and the implant is released from the delivery catheter. Patients may return to normal activities once the groin wound is determined to be secure.

CLINICAL RESULTS

Early clinical trials with the CardioSEAL® device focused on use for atrial septal defect. CardioSEAL® was quite effective in the small (<15 mm) defect with closure rates of 96% or greater at six months. STARFlex® results were similar in the ASD population. Tables 10.1–10.3 show the immediate and long-term results of the most frequent devices used to close these interatrial communications.

Evan M Zahn MD from Miami Children's Hospital, Miami, Florida, reported the initial results from a multi-center North American clinical trial for use of the CardioSEAL® for transcatheter closure of isolated secundum atrial septal defects in patients considered to be candidates for open heart surgical repair. Of 82 patients implanted with the CardioSEAL®, 96% achieved a clinically successful result. Dr Zahn concluded that these preliminary data suggested that the CardioSEAL® is a safe and effective device for transcatheter ASD closure. Kathy J Jenkins MD reported on the initial experience with CardioSEAL® for transcatheter closure of complex cardiac defects in high-risk patients in a study sponsored by Children's Hospital in Boston. Patients enter the trial following the determination by an independent medical review committee that they are at high risk of morbidity/mortality if treated surgically. Dr Jenkins reported on 117 patients implanted with 162 CardioSEAL® devices between May 1996 and August 1997 for a variety of cardiac defects, including ASD, ventricular septal defects, patent foramen ovale (PFO), and fenestrated Fontan operations. Dr Jenkins concluded that the findings suggest that the CardioSEAL® occluder device is an important alternative to surgery for high-risk patients. These findings reported at the American Heart Association meeting suggested both the effectiveness of the CardioSEAL® and the potential versatility of the device for a variety of clinical applications. Further investigations of the device are ongoing in North America. However, the CardioSEAL® is commercially available in most countries elsewhere in the world.

In the late 1990s, the focus of clinical use for these devices shifted to the PFO stroke TIA patient, in whom substantially more clinical reports are found. In general, PFO closure with both CardioSEAL® and STARFlex® is highly effective at the procedure level, with closure rates reported in the 98–99% range. Efficacy of PFO closure to prevent recurrent stroke or TIA is reported between 0% and 2.5% per year; however, these data are observational, and retrospective in nature.[5,7,8,12,16,17] The CLOSURE I trial will provide prospective, randomized data on efficacy in these patients. PFO closure has also been advocated for selected refractory migraine patients, based on observations that stroke patients with migraine history who had their PFOs closed for stroke prevention had dramatic decreases in headache frequency. In some reports, up to 50% or more of patients reported complete resolution of their headaches.[29] As with the stroke reports, these data are not prospectively collected in a randomized trial, hence are subject to criticism. However, the MIST trials have been designed to address the limitations of the observational reports. MIST I & II are well powered, randomized, prospective, double blind trials designed in conjunction with the migraine and cardiology communities. Results from MIST I are imminent at the time of writing.

Complications with NMT devices are very rare, and usually medically manageable.[4,15] Major complications include transient arrhythmia, vessel damage, embolization, and thrombus formation. Implant framework fracture, commonly reported in the early Clamshell years, is rarely reported with the modern implants. Importantly, patients with Clamshell devices implanted in the late 1980s and early 1990s that have had framework fractures documented, continue to do well. Complications from framework fracture are extremely rare (personal correspondence James Lock MD). Cardiac erosion, with and without tamponade, is a very rare event with NMT devices. Only one report exists in the literature.[18] Erosions, which are reported with some frequency with other devices, are less likely with NMT devices as the main framework is not made from shape memory materials (nitinol), thus facilitating excellent conformance of the implant to the variations in septal anatomy.

REFERENCES

1. Bush DM, Jenkins KH, Lock JE et al. Use of STARFlex Occlusion device reduces residual flow compared with CardioSEAL in the management of patent foramen ovale. Supplement to Circulation 2001; 104(17):II–746.
2. Anzai H, Child J, Natterson B et al. Incidence of thrombus formation on the CardioSEAL and the Amplatzer Interatrial Closure Devices. Am J Cardiol 2004; 93:426–31.
3. Krumsdorf U, Ostermayer S, Billinger K et al. Incidence and clinical course of thrombus formation on atrial septal defect and patient foramen ovale closure devices in 1,000 constructive patients. J Am Coll Cardiol 2004; 43(2):302–9.
4. Alameddine, F, Block, PC. Transcatheter patent foramen ovale closure for secondary prevention of paradoxical embolic events: Acute results from the FORECAST Registry. Cathet Cardiovasc Interventions 2004; 62:512–16.
5. Martin F, Sanchez PL, Doherty E et al. Percutaneous transcatheter closure of patent foramen ovela in patients with paradoxical embolism. Circulation 2002; 106:1121–6.
6. Butera G, Bini MR, Chessa M, Bedogni F, Onofri M, Carminati M. Transcatheter closure of patent foramen ovale in patients with cryptogenic stroke. Ital Heart J 2001; 2(2):115–8.
7. Khairy P, O'Donnell CP, Landzberg MJ. Transcatheter closure versus medical therapy of patent foramen ovale and presumed paradoxical thromboemboli, a systematic review. Ann Intern Med 2003; 139:753–60.
8. Meier B, Lock JE. Contemporary management of patent foramen ovale. Circulation 2003; 107(1):5–9.
9. Reisman M, Gray WA, Olsen JV. Relief of migraine headaches associated with closure of patent foramen ovale. J Am Coll Cardiol 2003; 19:41(6) Supplement A:474A.
10. Reisman M, Jesurum J, Spencer M et al. Migraine relief following transcatheter closure of patent foramen ovale. J Am Coll Cardiol 2004; 3:43 (5) Supplement A:376A.
11. Reisman M, Chrisofferson RD, Jesurum J et al. Migraine headache relief after transcatheter closure of patent foramen ovale. J Am Coll Cardiol 2005; 45: 493–5.
12. Rhodes JF, Abouk-Chebl A, Lane GK et al. CardioSEAL transcatheter patent foramen ovale closure after acute embolic neurologic events. Am J Cardiol 2002; 90(suppl 6A): 37H.
13. Sievert et al. Transcatheter closure of patent foramen ovale for prevention of paradoxical embolism and recurrent embolic stroke with the CardioSEAL STARFlex occluder. Am J Cardiol 2002; 90(suppl 6A): 38H.

14. Sommer RJ, Kramer PH, Sorensen SG et al. Closure of patent foramen ovale with CardioSEAL septal occluder: highly effective intervention. Am J Cardiol 2002; 90(suppl 6A): 37H.
15. Sommer RJ, Kramer PH, Sorensen SG et al. Closure of patent foramen ovale with CardioSEAL septal occluder: A safe intervention. Am J Cardiol 2002; 90(suppl 6A): 136H.
16. Sommer RJ, Kramer PH, Sorensen SG et al. Closure of patent foramen ovale with CardioSEAL septal occluder: infrequent recurrent thrombotic neurologic events. Am J Cardiol 2002; 90(suppl 6A): 136H.
17. Varma C, Benson LN, Warr MR et al. Clinical outcomes of patent foramen ovale closure for paradoxical emboli without echocardiographic guidance. Cathet Cardiovasc Interventions 2004; 62:519–25.
18. Pinto FF, Sousa L, Fragata J. Late cardiac tamponade after transcatheter closure of atrial septal defect with CardioSEAL® device. Cardiol Young 2001; 11(2):233–5.
19. Fischer G, Stieh J, Uebing A, Hoffmann U, Morf G, Kramer HH. Experience with transcatheter closure of secundum atrial septal defects using the Amplatzer septal occluder: a single centre study in 236 consecutive patients. Heart 2003 Feb; 89(2):199–204.
20. Omeish A, Hijazi ZM. Transcatheter closure of atrial septal defects in children & adults using the Amplatzer Septal Occluder. Interv Cardiol 2001 Feb; 14(1):37–44.
21. Du ZD, Hijazi ZM, Kleinman CS, Silverman NH, Larntz K. Amplatzer investigators comparison between transcatheter and surgical closure of secundum atrial septal defect in children and adults: results of a multicenter nonrandomized trial. J Am Coll Cardiol 2002; 39(11):1836–44.
22. Rickers C, Hamm C, Stern H et al. Percutaneous closure of secundum atrial septal defect with a new self centereing device ("angel wings"). Heart 1998; 80:517–21.
23. El-Said HG, Bezold LI, Grifka RG et al. Sizing of Atrial septal defects to predict successful C Transcatheter CardioSEAL Device. Tex Heart Inst J 2001; 28:177–82.
24. Reisman M, Christofferson RD, Jesurum J et al. Migraine headache relief after transcatheter closure of patent foramen ovale. J Am Coll Cardiol 2005; 45:493–5.
25. Varma Ch, Benson LN, Warr MR et al. Clinical outcomes of patent foramen ovale closure for paradoxical emboli without echocardiographic guidance. Catheter Cardiovasc Interv 2004; 62:519–25.
26. Hung J, Landzberg MJ, Jenkins KJ et al. Closure of patent foramen ovale for paradoxical emboli: Intermediate-term risk of recurrent neurological events following transcatheter device placement. J Am Coll of Cardiol 2000; 35:1311–16.
27. Kreutzer J, Ryan CA, Wright JA et al. Acute animal studies of the STARFlex system: A new self-centering CardioSEAL septal occluder. Cathet Cardiovasc Intervent 2000; 49:225–33.
28. Bialkowski J, Kusa J, Szkutnik M et al. Percutaneous closure of atrial septal dfefect. Short term and mid-term results. Rev Esp Cardiol 2003; 56:383–8.
29. Butera G, Carminati M, Chesa M et al. CardioSEAL/STARTFlex versus Amplatzer devices for percutaneous closure of small to moderate (up to 18 mm) atrial septal defects. Am Heart J 2004; 148:507–10.
30. Knebel F, Gliech V, Walde T et al. Percutaneous closure of interatrial communications in the prospective embolism prevention study with two and three dimensional echocardiography. Cardiovascular Ultrasound 2004; 2:5.
31. Herrmann HC, Silvestry FE, Glaser R et al. Percutaneous patent foramen ovale and atrial septal defect closure in adults: Results and device comparison in 100 consecutive implants at single center. Catheter Cardiovasc Interv 2005; 64:197–203.
32. Rao PS. Results of transvenous occlusion of secundum atrial septal defects. Argentine Federation of Cardiology 2001.
33. Tuzcu V, Michel-Behnke I, Schranz D. Transcatheter closure of atrial septal defects: Expetience of a pediatric heart center. Euro J Gen Med 2004; 1:33–6.

11

The Premere* PFO occluder

Horst Sievert and Franziska Büscheck

Introduction • The device • Implantation procedure

INTRODUCTION

Devices able to close atrial septal defects percutaneously were developed in the 1980s, and these devices have been used subsequently to close PFOs as well.[1] As they were originally developed to close true atrial septal defects, devices currently used to close PFOs have certain characteristics in common, such as right and left atrial anchor arms that are rigidly connected to each other at a fixed distance, and a means to physically close tissue defects ('umbrella' fabric design or extensive metal strutwork to encourage tissue overgrowth).

Unlike an ASD, however, a PFO is a 'tunnel' with a variable length but without a tissue defect. The tunnel length can vary from 2 mm up to as much as 20 mm, and the right and left atrial openings of the tunnel may be offset from each other. Furthermore, the septum itself has a variable thickness, resulting in right and left atrial septal walls that are not parallel to one another. The Premere device was specifically designed to accommodate these PFO and septal characteristics (Figure 11.1).

It is a percutaneous, transcatheter, self-expanding dual-anchor arm occlusion device that is made of nickel-titanium alloy (nitinol). The currently available sizes are 20 or 25 mm in diameter. The device consists of two flexible anchors connected via an adjustable length tether made of polyester. The left atrial anchor is made without fabric, so it has less foreign material in the left side of the heart. It has an open architecture, a low profile, and a small surface area which potentially minimize the risk of thrombus formation and the potential for atrial tissue erosion. Only the right anchor is enveloped between two layers of knitted polyester fabric. Both anchors are designed with a low surface and low profile area to assist a rapid endothelialization and minimize exposure to thrombogenic surfaces.

The flexible polyester braided tether runs through the center of the anchor and holds both together. It allows a variable distance between the anchors in order to adjust to the anatomy. The tether length permits the right and left arms

*Premere is a registered trade mark of St. Jude Medical Inc, Maple Grove, MN.

to pivot freely with regard to one another, and to conform to any variations in septal thickness. These features also allow the anchors to be placed directly across each opening of the tunnel with minimal distortion to the septal anatomy. The anchors are locked together after delivery and then the tether is cut.

The schematic of the implant portion of the PFO closure device with the delivery system is depicted in Figure 11.2.

In November 2003 the first Premere PFO device was implanted in our center. Since then PFO closure using this occluder has been performed in over 100 patients successfully.

THE DEVICE

The left atrial anchor consists of four radiating clover-leaf-like arms. A radiopaque outer marker rivet is placed at the ends of each arm.

At the center of the anchor a radiopaque left-side hub is permanently fixed to the left anchor and the tether.

The right atrial anchor is similar to the left one. It has also a right-side hub marker which is longer than that of the left anchor and has a flange to allow for retrieval if needed. In addition, the nitinol anchor is enclosed within the right-side covering made of polyester. This material is a PET material that is

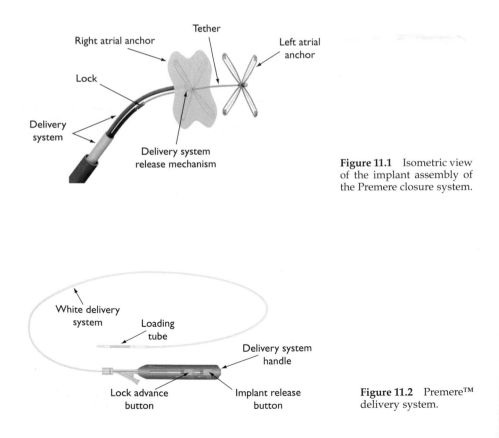

Figure 11.1   Isometric view of the implant assembly of the Premere closure system.

Figure 11.2   Premere™ delivery system.

commonly used in vascular prosthesis. The right atrial anchor rides freely on the tether in both directions for ease of advancement and retrieval.

The implant assembly consists of the right and the left atrium anchor. Both are kept together by a mechanism that locks onto the tether on the proximal side of the right atrial anchor.

A cross-section of the complete implant assembly is shown in Figure 11.3.

The tether is a braided white polyester (PET) suture-like material. The tether termination engages with the left-side hub marker of the left atrial anchor. Near the proximal end of the tether there is a marker to denote the position to move the tether retention clip to after the deployment of the left anchor. On the proximal side of the right atrial anchor the tether is trimmed after the anchors and lock are in place.

The tether lock is made up of nitinol tubing with six tabs which are placed on two circumferential planes. The tether runs through the center of the lock. The tabs are designed to dig into the tether so that it is movable in one direction only.

The tether lock is encased with a lock marker. It is made of platinum-iridium alloy that makes the tether lock visible under fluoroscopy.

A tether cutter system is advanced over the tether after the delivery catheter system is removed. It is made of an outer and an inner cutter shaft. To advance the outer cutter shaft forward, an outer cutter hub is rotated clockwise (Figure 11.4). This mechanism cuts the tether as it is pushed against the wall of the tether guide lumen.

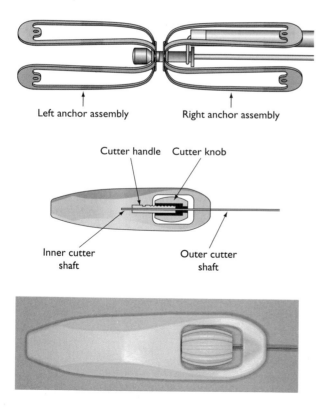

Left anchor assembly   Right anchor assembly

Figure 11.3 Implant assembly in the pre-loaded state.

Cutter handle   Cutter knob

Inner cutter shaft   Outer cutter shaft

Figure 11.4 Tether cutter hub (proximal).

The guide catheter is available in two distal curve shapes in order to provide a better accommodation to the different anatomies of the patients. The two curves of the guide catheter are:

- 25 degree radius of curvature
- 45 degree radius of curvature.

Except for the radius of curvature of the distal tip the two guide catheters are identical. They consist of an obturator which is a proximal hub with a standard side arm for flushing. The schematic of the guide catheter is shown in Figure 11.5.

All patients received aspirin and clopidogrel the day of the implantation, and were heparinized during the procedure to an ACT of at least 250 seconds. Fluoroscopy and echocardiography were used as per the operator's preference. Prophylactic antibiotic treatment, i.e., administration of an intravenous first-generation cephalosporin, was recommended before and after the procedure.

IMPLANTATION PROCEDURE

The right femoral vein is punctured, the 11F introducer sheath is placed and the dilator/obturator is loaded into the blue Premere delivery sheath.

The blue delivery sheath and dilator/obturator are advanced along the guide-wire into the right atrium, through the PFO and into the left atrium.

The dilator/obturator and delivery sheath should not advance in the absence of a guide-wire.

The guide-wire is removed. Care should be taken that the tip of the delivery sheath is in the mid-left atrium and is neither obstructed nor in contact with tissue. The dilator/obturator hub is kept below atrial level, blood should flow freely out of the hub. The dilator/obturator is slowly removed while a constant column of blood out of the proximal end of the dilator/obturator is maintained.

The delivery sheath is flushed with heparizined saline.

Pressure is maintained on the syringe, and the loading tube is advanced into the hub until its shoulder fits correctly against the hub of the delivery sheath.

The implant assembly is transferred into the delivery sheath by slowly advancing the Premere PFO closure system at least 5 cm into the delivery sheath.

The Premere implant is advanced through the blue delivery sheath until the implant is near the distal tip of the delivery sheath. This should be done under fluoroscopic guidance.

The left atrial anchor is deployed by slowly advancing the white delivery system. This occurs until the radiopaque markers on the tips of the left atrial anchor arms expand and move away from each other (Figures 11.6a and 11.6b).

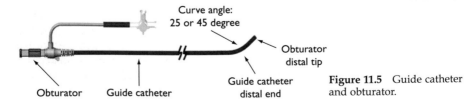

Figure 11.5 Guide catheter and obturator.

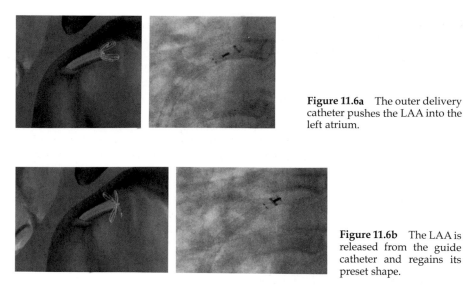

Figure 11.6a The outer delivery catheter pushes the LAA into the left atrium.

Figure 11.6b The LAA is released from the guide catheter and regains its preset shape.

Once the left anchor is deployed, the right hand is placed on the mark located on the tether of the Premere PFO closure system. The tether is used to maintain tactile feeling of the septum and to direct device placement.

Slight tension is applied to the tether to maintain the orientation of the left atrial anchor perpendicular to the end of the delivery sheath. Both the delivery sheath and tether are slowly retracted until the left anchor is securely seated against the septal wall.

Retraction of the blue delivery sheath into the mid-right atrium is continued. While retracting the delivery sheath the white delivery system will slide back over the fixed tether (Figures 11.7a and 11.7b).

The position of the delivery sheath in the right atrium is verified under fluoroscopy. While maintaining slight tension on the tether, the right atrial anchor is slowly advanced out of the blue delivery sheath by advancing the white delivery system. Advancing of the right anchor is continued until it is seated against the septal wall of the right atrium.

If necessary, repositioning of the right anchor is possible by retracting the white delivery system and re-advancing it. To direct the right atrial anchor into the desired location tension is used on the tether (Figures 11.8a and 11.8b).

Care should be taken to ensure that the right atrial anchor is not advanced into the PFO track. Ensure that the anchor arms do not constrain or prolapse into the PFO tunnel.

The touhy borst on the Premere delivery system is loosened while tension is maintained on the tether. The inner delivery catheter is advanced. This movement will push the lock mechanism forward. Advancing of the lock mechanism is continued until the radiopaque marker on the lock mechanism is adjacent to the radiopaque marker on the right-side anchor (Figure 11.9). This should be done under fluoroscopic guidance.

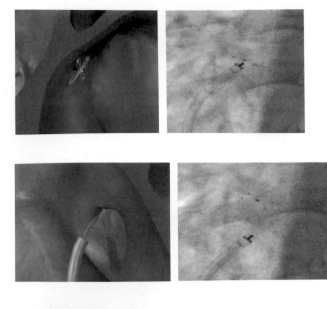

Figure 11.7a The guide catheter with the LAA in slight tension is withdrawn and the arms of the LAA draw the PFO flap towards the atrial septum.

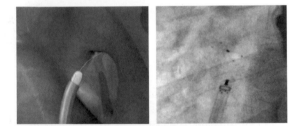

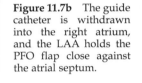

Figure 11.7b The guide catheter is withdrawn into the right atrium, and the LAA holds the PFO flap close against the atrial septum.

Figure 11.8a The delivery catheter system pushes the RAA out of the guide catheter into the right atrium.

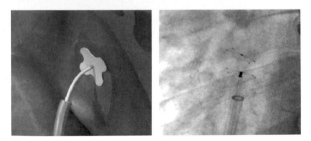

Figure 11.8b The delivery catheter system pushes the RAA against the septum secundum of the right atrium.

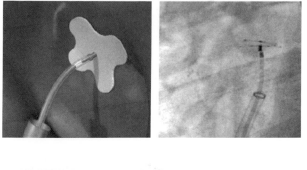

Figure 11.9a The distance between the RAA and LAA is adjusted until flush with the septum. The tether lock is advanced over the tether with the inner delivery catheter to lock the position of the LAA and RAA.

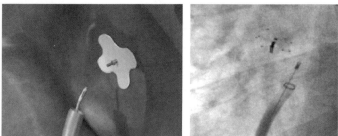

Figure 11.9b The tether is cut by the tether cutter system.

The Premere delivery system is retracted into the tip of the guide catheter. The tether needs to be pulled to ensure that the implant is securely in place. This should be observed under fluoroscopy at a minimum. The tether retention clip button must then be depressed and held while it is slid proximally off the tether together with the Premere delivery system. The proximal end of the tether is introduced into the distal end of the cutter and the tether is advanced until it exits the cutter. Slight rotation of the tether may be required to advance it through the proximal opening of the cutter. Tension is maintained on the tether and the cutter is advanced into the proximal end of the guide catheter until the radiopaque marker on the cutter is adjacent to the radiopaque marker on the lock mechanism. This should also be observed under fluoroscopy.

While maintaining tension on the tether the cutter wheel is rotated clockwise (typically four turns) until the tether has been cut. This will be observed by a change in tension on the tether and typically by a change in position of the radiopaque marker of the cutter relative to the radiopaque marker on the lock mechanism. The cutter wheel is rotated counter clockwise to its original position. The cutter and the cut tether are removed together out of the guide catheter.

It is recommended that a right atriogram at a minimum of three orthogonal angles is performed to document the position of the implant relative to the atrial anatomy.

Finally the Premere guide catheter is removed (Figures 11.10a and 11.10b).

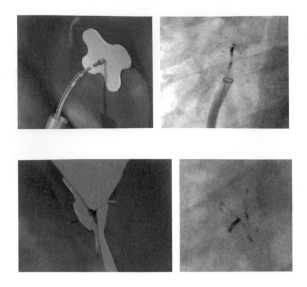

Figure 11.10a The Delivery catheter system is withdrawn from the guide catheter and the tether cutter system guided to the implant site by the tether.

Figure 11.10b PFO closed by the implant assembly.

Premere retrieval basket

The Velocimed Premere retrieval basket is a percutaneous, transcatheter, self-expanding, retrieval device. The retrieval basket consists of funnel-shaped mesh of braided nitinol wire that is mechanically crimped to a stainless steel shaft. The shaft is long enough to allow the basket to be advanced out of the distal tip of the Premere delivery sheath.

How to use

The Premere retrieval basket is indicated for use in extracting a Premere PFO closure system implant that has been deployed incorrectly into the right or left atrium of the heart. The Premere retrieval basket is only required in the event that both the right and left atrial anchors have been inadvertently placed in the same atrium.

Procedure

Prior to use, a 20 ml syringe filled with heparinized saline solution is attached to the Luer fitting on the carrier tube. The carrier tube and the retrieval basket are flushed until all of the air is evacuated out of the loading tube.

To use the Premere retrieval basket, the Premere PFO closure system delivery catheter must be removed, and the tether must not have been cut. The tether is inserted into the eye of the tether threading tool. The free end of the tether is held while the tether threading tool is retracted through the retrieval basket and the loading tube. This should be done until the tether threading tool and the tether exit the opposite side of the loading tube. The tether is released and removed and the tether threading tool is discarded.

Tension should be applied to the proximal end of the tether and the loading tube is inserted into the delivery sheath. Adequate time should allow for blood to completely fill the loading tube. The retrieval basket is advanced into the delivery sheath and the loading tube is slid out of the delivery sheath. The retrieval basket is advanced to the distal tip of the delivery sheath such that the funnel extends beyond the tip of the delivery sheath and expands into the atrium (Figure 11.11).

The retrieval basket should be observed with fluoroscopy and ultrasound when advancing to the desired location.

The implant assembly is pulled into the basket with the tether until it is completely seated at the bottom of the funnel-shaped basket. Both the tether and shaft of the basket are pulled together until the implant is withdrawn into the delivery sheath and completely removed.

Post-interventional treatment and follow-up examinations

Patients are discharged on a regimen of 100 mg/day aspirin as well as 75 mg/day of clopidogrel over six months. A sub-acute bacterial endocarditis prophylaxis is recommended for six months after implant as well. Patients should have been seen for follow-up visits at two weeks, three months and six months post-implant. A bubble study is required at the two week follow-up visit and at each scheduled follow-up visit until complete closure of the PFO is demonstrated.

The Close-up study showed that the Premere device was safely implanted in all cases, and provided complete closure of the PFO in 87% of the cases at six months. Closure rate was clearly related to the device size. The 20 mm device had a better closure rate than the 15 mm device that was only available initially.

No serious device-related adverse events occurred during implantation or at follow-up. One patient had two single episodes of atrial fibrillation which had resolved by four months post implant. Although one patient reported transient left arm weakness, he did not seek medical attention at the time, and no work-up was able to be done. This patient had no evidence of device thrombus at any evaluation and the PFO was found to be closed on echo/bubble study.

Braun et al[2] reported their results in 307 consecutive patients with symptomatic PFO using three different devices (PFO-Star, Amplatzer® PFO Occluder,

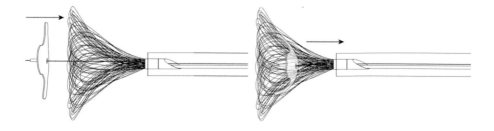

Figure 11.11 Pulling the implant into the retrieval basket.

and CardioSEAL®/STARFlex®). They were able to implant the chosen device successfully in every case and reported peri-interventional complications in nine patients.

In a study of 66 patients, Bruch et al were able to successfully implant a PFO closure device in every intended patient with no complications during the procedure.[3]

These data as well as the data from the Close-up trial indicate that closure of PFO can be successfully and safely completed.

In a study of 1,000 consecutive patients, Krumdorf et al reported thrombus formation in 5/407 ASD patients and in 15 of 593 PFO patients at four weeks and six months after implantation.[4] In a recent case history, Ruge et al report a left atrial thrombus on a STARFlex® device three years after implantation.[5]

In the Close-up study, where transesophageal echocardiograms were performed that included a detailed examination of the left atrial anchor for evidence of thrombus, no patients were found to have device-related thrombus at any time.

These data demonstrate that the Premere device can safely and effectively close PFO. Further studies should be undertaken to demonstrate the effectiveness of PFO closure with the Premere in reducing the incidence of thrombo-embolic events such as cryptogenic stroke.

REFERENCES

1. Sievert H, Horvath K, Zadan E et al. Patent foramen ovale closure in patients with transient ischemic attack/stroke. J Interv Cardiol 2001; 14(2):261–6.
2. Braun M, Gliech V, Boscheri A, Schoen S et al. Transcatheter closure of patent foramen ovale (PFO) in patients with paradoxical embolism. Eur Heart J 2004; 25:424–30.
3. Bruch L, Parsi A, Grad MO et al. Transcatheter closure of interatrial communications for secondary prevention of paradoxical embolism. Circulation 2002; 105:2845–8.
4. Krumsdorf U, Ostermayer S, Billinger K et al. Incidence and clinical course of thrombus formation on atrial septal defect and patent foramen ovale closure devices in 1000 consecutive patients. J Am Coll Cardiol 2004; 43:302–9.
5. Ruge H, Wildhirt SM, Libera P et al. Left atrial thrombus on atrial septal defect closure device as a source of cerebral emboli 3 years after implantation. Circulation 2005; 112:e130–1.

12

The Cardia-Intrasept PFO closure device

Rainer Schräder

Introduction • Device description • Component description • Animal testing
• Technique for transcatheter PFO closure • Clinical results of transcatheter PFO
closure • Conclusion

INTRODUCTION

The anatomy of the atrial septum is extremely variable. In patients with patent foramen ovale (PFO), the size of the defect may be as small as 2 mm on the one hand and as large as 2 cm on the other. The length of the PFO channel may be as short as 2 mm and as long as 10 mm. The thickness of the septum secundum may vary between 3 and 12 mm and variable redundancy of tissue may be the reason for a mobile, hypermobile, or aneurysmal septum primum.

DEVICE DESCRIPTION

The Intrasept device is a transcatheter PFO-closure device that has been designed to accommodate these anatomical variations of the interatrial communication by means of a flexible (in all three dimensions) connection between the left- and right-atrial sails of the occluder (Figures 12.1 and 12.2).

The device consists of two sails of white, polyvinyl alcohol foam (PVA) attached to a nitinol and titanium frame. The frame itself is comprised of a double articulating centerpost with radiating stranded nitinol wire struts, each with a small titanium endcap. The nitinol struts secure the device in place, holding each PVA sail on its respective side of the interatrial septum. The PVA sails close to the patent foramen ovale by compressing the overlapping septum primum and septum secundum together in a 'closed' position.

The device provides a scaffolding on which endothelial in-growth will occur. This in-growth combined with the frame of the device also effectively stabilizes the atrial septum including those with aneurysm. At the right atrial side of the centerpost is a grasping knob where the delivery forceps attaches to hold and subsequently release the device during implantation (Figure 12.3 shows a schematic view of the Intrasept device).

The unique design of the centerpost allows each sail to articulate independently through 360 degrees. The sails are thus able to conform to their respective

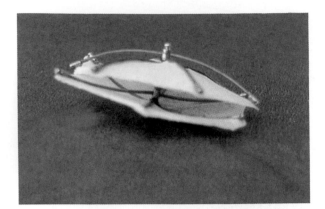

Figure 12.1   Intrasept device.

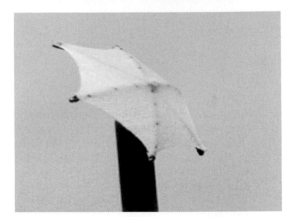

Figure 12.2   Intrasept device during deployment.

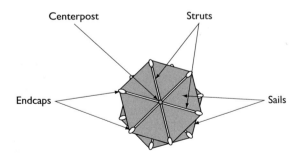

Figure 12.3   Components of the Intrasept device.

atrial anatomy in a flat profile. Seating of the device within the defect automatically occurs in a configuration which produces the least amount of mechanical stress on both the device as well as the surrounding tissue. This serves to minimize or eliminate a variety of possible complications including tissue trauma and necrosis, perforation, device fracture, and embolization (Figures 12.4 and 12.5).

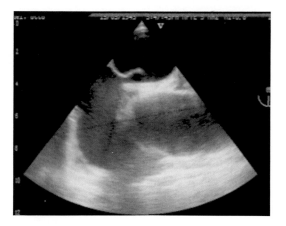

Figure 12.4   Patent foramen ovale with atrial septum aneurysm.

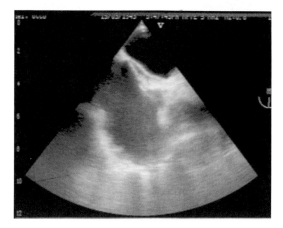

Figure 12.5   Implanted Intrasept device stabilizing the septal aneurysm.

COMPONENT DESCRIPTION

Sail(s): There are two sails of identical size on each device made of polyvinyl alcohol foam (PVA) which is natural in color (white). The sails vary in diagonal size from 20–35 mm to accommodate a wide range of PFO defects. Sails are attached to the struts with polypropylene suture. The left atrial sail is attached over the left struts while the right atrial sail is attached under the right struts.

Struts: Struts consist of 19 individual strands of nitinol and are constructed in a manner which maximizes fatigue resistance while still maintaining appropriate physiological tension. They provide structure and definition for the sails of the device and vary in length from 20–35 mm according to the size of the device manufactured.

End caps: End caps are milled from solid titanium and are mechanically crimped to the ends of the struts. The end caps serve as an anchor point for suturing the sails to the struts and further provide a 'soft' end on each arm of the device eliminating the potential for tissue damage caused by the ends of the struts.

Centerpost: The Intrasept centerpost is constructed of titanium using a patented double articulating multi-joint system (Figure 12.6). This arrangement is unique in that it allows each sail to move independently from the other in all three dimensions. The sails are thus able to conform precisely to the defect anatomy without stenting the PFO open, and the device automatically seats itself in the position which produces the least amount of stress on the struts and surrounding tissue. The right side of the centerpost includes a grasping knob for attachment of the delivery forceps.

Delivery forceps: The Intrasept system includes a flexible delivery forceps with jaws to grab and to release the device at the grasping knob during deployment and retrieval, if necessary. The forceps handle provides a locking mechanism, which prevents detachment of the Intrasept, allowing a controlled release of the device only when ready. The handle of the forceps is constructed from #303 stainless steel and the spool and thumb ring are acetal copolymer.

The shaft of the forceps is also constructed from #303 stainless steel and consists of a central rod surrounded by a flexible coil. The last 10 cm of the forceps is flat ground to provide flexibility.

The jaws are ASTM A564, type 630 stainless steel. These are mechanically pinned and welded to the shaft mechanism of the forceps to provide the necessary opening and closing action. The jaws have a hole in the end that corresponds to the size of the grasping knob on the centerpost of the Intrasept (Figure 12.7).

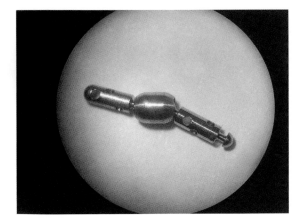

Figure 12.6 Intrasept titanium centerpost.

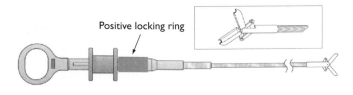

Positive locking ring

Figure 12.7 Intrasept delivery forceps.

Loading sheath: The loading sheath is a short, flared-tip tube made of fluorinated ethylene propylene (FEP) that is transparent blue in color. Its dimensions are approximately 0.20 inch diameter by 2.80 inches length with a 0.35 inch diameter flare thermally formed at one end. The loading sheath serves as an aid to properly fold the Intrasept for transfer into the delivery sheath (Figure 12.8).

All device component materials (Table 12.1) have a long history of use in medical device applications, and have been well characterized for their physical properties and biocompatibility. The Intrasept device is MRI compatible and additional models are available for transcatheter closure of ASD, PDA, fenestrated Fontan, and a variety of other defects (Table 12.2).

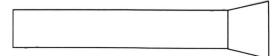

Figure 12.8 Intrasept loading sheath.

Table 12.1 Component materials

Device	Component	Material
Intrasept device	Foam sails	Polyvinyl alcohol (Ivalon®)
	Centerpost	Titanium
	Struts	Titanium-nickel alloy (Nitinol)
	Sutures	Polypropylene
	Adhesive	Class VI cyanoacrylate
	End caps	Titanium
Intrasept delivery forceps	Shaft	Stainless steel
	Jaws	Stainless steel
Intrasept loading sheath	Loading sheath	FEP (fluorinated ethylene propylene)

Table 12.2 Device size and model numbers

Model number	Centerpost (length, mm)	PVA sail (diagonal length in mm)
PFO-320A	3	20
PFO-325A	3	25
PFO-330A	3	30
PFO-335A	3	35

ANIMAL TESTING

Initially, animal implant testing of the Cardia Intrasept Device (precursor) was performed to verify feasibility and efficacy. The objective of the study was to demonstrate effective closure of the open foramen ovale and endothelialization of the device with favorable tissue compatibility. The study was performed over a period of 131 days using Merino sheep with persistent foramen ovale accomplished via interventional balloon dilation.

Implantation of the device was achieved in all subjects. Clinical tests were performed at 1, 7, and 14 days after implantation and catheter tests done 7 to 131 days after implantation showed correct placement of the implants with no coronary insufficiencies. Macroscopic post-mortem tests did not indicate any inflammatory changes of the coronary valves, perforations, or obstructions of pulmonary veins or the coronary sinus. A complete covering of the PVA foam sails with a whitish translucent tissue was visible after only 29 days with a transition from thrombus formation to fibro-muscular integration occurring. After 53 days the entire implant was completely covered and at 131 days the fibro-muscular ingrowth was complete with several giant cells visible. A histological analysis did not show any inflammation or foreign body reaction to the implant (Figures 12.9 and 12.10).

The study concluded with no acute or chronic symptoms of inflammation within a period of up to 131 days after implantation. The device was completely integrated both macroscopically and microscopically after only 53 days and was thus effective for occlusion of the PFO without adverse tissue reaction.

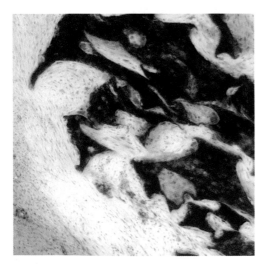

Figure 12.9   Histology at 47 days.

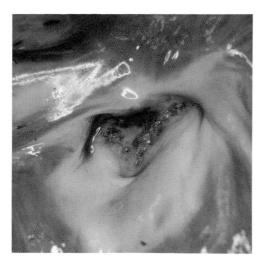

Figure 12.10 Right atrial in-growth at 47 days.

TECHNIQUE FOR TRANSCATHETER PFO CLOSURE

Techniques may vary between different hospitals and individual operators. In the author's opinion, echocardiographic (transvenous, transesophageal, or, in some cases, transthoracic) guidance is helpful in most patients while balloon-sizing of the PFO is not required in the vast majority of cases. This is a proposal for a simple and safe procedure that requires 20–30 minutes on the catheterization table and 18–36 hours in the hospital (including day 1 follow-up).

Premedication: Aspirin (100 mg) and clopidogrel (300 mg) should be started the day before implantation. At the day of implantation, one to three standard doses of a second-generation cephalosporin or ampicillin for prophylaxis of bacterial endocarditis should be administered. After sheath placement into the right femoral vein, heparin is administered as 100 units unfractioned heparin per kg bodyweight. After premedication with 0.5–1.0 mg atropine, 10 mg metoclopramide, and sedatives as required the transesophageal echo probe is introduced.

Procedure: A 5 French multipurpose catheter can be used for angiography of the fossa ovalis (Figure 12.11). This visualizes the anatomy of the septum primum and the septum secundum as well as the length and the orientation of the PFO channel. After crossing the septum, the tip of the catheter is placed into the anterior left pulmonary vein and the position checked by injection of a small amount of contrast medium. The multipurpose catheter is exchanged for a 10–12 French transseptal sheath by means of an extra stiff 0.035-inch exchange wire.

Thereafter, angiography of the left atrium can be performed in order to determine the size and shape of the atrium and the atrial septum, especially in patients who do not tolerate the transesophageal echo probe. The selected (selection may be based on echocardiographic data) device is then delivered through the transseptal sheath under fluoroscopic as well as transesophageal echocardiographic guidance. Care should be taken to remove any air bubbles from the loading system as well as from the sheath. The distal (left-atrial) part of the

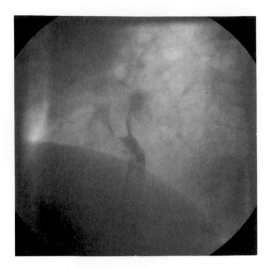

Figure 12.11   Angiography of the fossa ovalis.

device is opened and pulled back together with delivery system and sheath against the septum. This can be felt as an elastic resistance with pulse-synchronous movements of the occluder. It is difficult, but not impossible, to inadvertently pull the device through the septum. By keeping slight tension on the delivery system, the sheath is then pulled back until the proximal (right atrial) part of the occluder opens. Before and after release, the position of the device can be checked by right atrial contrast injection through the transseptal sheath (Figure 12.12).

Postinterventional treatment and follow-up: Usually, patients can be discharged from the hospital the next day. Before discharge, white blood cell count and C-reactive protein are measured. The position of the device is confirmed by chest X-ray and transthoracic echocardiography. For the prophylaxis of

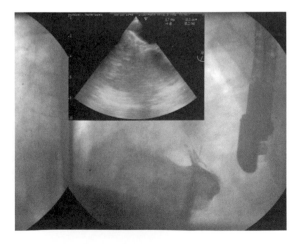

Figure 12.12   Post-implant right atriogram.

thrombembolic events after device implantation, patients are treated with 75 mg clopidogrel for four weeks and with 100 mg aspirin for six months. Standard bacterial endocarditis prophylaxis is recommended for 12 months. After six months, transesophageal contrast echocardiography should be performed for detection of residual shunting. Thereafter, patients are followed annually either by telephone contact or by their referring physicians.

CLINCAL RESULTS OF TRANSCATHETER PFO CLOSURE

Patients: From June 2002 until October 2005 transcatheter PFO closure with an Intrasept device was attempted in 189 patients (85 women and 104 men), aged 21–77 (mean, 52.7) years. Among these, 95 patients (50%) also had an atrial septal aneurysm (ASA). Deep venous thrombosis was found by either phlebography or Doppler ultrasonography with frequency analysis and B-mode in 17 patients (9%) and 4 patients (2%) had had pulmonary embolism. Before PFO closure, the patients had suffered a total of 284 embolic events of whom 194 (68%) were strokes, 85 (30%) were transient ischemic attacks, and 5 (2%) were peripheral embolism. Individual patients had experienced 1 to 3 events with an average of 1.5 events per patient. The incidence of embolic events before PFO closure was 2.9%/year (284 events in 9960 patient-years), 1.9%/year for stroke, and 1.0%/year for TIA and peripheral embolism.

Interventions: General anesthesia was not required and device implantation was performed with fluoroscopic guidance only in nine patients. Balloon-sizing of the PFO was not performed. The fluoroscopy time ranged from 0.7 to 7.1 min (median, 2.1 min), the duration of the procedure was from 15 to 60 min (median, 25 min), and the lenghth of hospital stay was shorter than 48 hours in >90% of patients. PFO closure was successful in all patients (at the first attempt in 186 patients and with a second device in three patients).

Transient ST-segment elevation was observed in two patients and in one patient partial misplacement of the device (five arms on the left side and seven arms on the right side of the atrial septum with stable overall position of the device) occurred due to incorrect loading of the occluder. There were no other serious complications, especially no neurologic deficits, no perforations, no myocardial infarctions, and no need for surgical interventions.

Follow-up: The total follow-up time is now 206 patient-years with a mean follow-up interval of 13 months (range, 0.5–3.3 years). No information is available for 17 patients (9%) while 118 of 141 eligible patients have completed the six months follow-up including chest X-ray and transesophageal contrast echocardiography. At six months follow-up, residual right-to-left shunting was detected in 13/118 patients (10.7%).

There were no thrombi detected by transesophageal echocardiography and no wire fractures observed with X-ray. In one patient, the occluder system was removed surgically during coronary bypass surgery six months after implantation, and in another after four weeks because of endocarditis following an accident leading to posttraumatic septicemia.

During the follow-up period, three patients had a total of four recurrent events (1.9%/year). The incidence of recurrent stroke (defined as neurologic symptoms and newly detected brain defect) was 1.4%/year and the incidence of recurrent TIA (defined as reversible neurologic symptoms but without brain defect) was 0.5%/year. None of these patients suffered a permanent neurologic deficit after PFO closure.

CONCLUSION

Over the past decade the association of cerebrovascular events and patent foramen ovale has been increasingly recognized with the passage of emboli through the foramen (i.e. paradoxical embolism) thought to be the underlying pathophysiological mechanism.[1–16] There are, so far, no randomized prospective data available comparing PFO closure with other therapeutic strategies (e.g. surgery, oral anticoagulation, antiplatelet therapy).[17]

The annual incidence of recurrent cerebrovascular events with medical therapy varies between 4% and 8%.[18–25] Device closure of PFO seems to yield better clinical results with reccurrence rates between 2% and 4% per year.[25–42] Clinical complications after device implantation include embolization, perforation, thrombus formation, wire fractures, and residual shunting.[43–46]

The preliminary clinical data with the Intrasept device presented here seem to be promising. The incidence of stroke or TIA was lower after transcatheter PFO closure (1.9%/year) as in the lifetime of these patients before the intervention (2.8%/year). Technical problems occurred only in a minority of patients, although 50% of these patients had an atrial septal aneurysm, an anatomic variation where device implantation is clearly more challenging than in patients with PFO alone.[47]

Therefore, transcatheter PFO closure with this newly developed device seems to be acceptable in selected patients after full explanation of the potential benefits and the potential risks. However, all patients undergoing PFO-device closure should be monitored prospectively for an unlimited period of time.

REFERENCES

1. Cohnheim J. In: Thrombose und Embolie: Vorlesung über allgemeine Pathologie. Berlin, Germany: Hirschwald, Berlin (Publishers); 1877:134.
2. Hart RG, Miller VT. Cerebral infarction in young adults: a practical approach. Stroke 1983; 14:110–14.
3. Hagen PT, Scholz DG, Edwards WD. Incidence and size of patent foramen ovale during the first 10 decades of life: an autopsy study of 965 normal hearts. Mayo Clin Proc 1984; 59:17–20.
4. Lechat P, Mas JL, Lascult G et al. Prevalence of patent foramen ovale in patients with stroke. New Engl J Med 1988; 318:1148–52.
5. De Belder MA, Tourikis L, Leech G, Camm AJ. Risk of patent foramen ovale for thromboembolic events in all age groups. Am J Cardiol 1992; 69:1316–20.
6. Hausmann D, Mügge A, Becht I, Daniel WG. Diagnosis of patent foramen ovale by transesophageal echocardiography and association with cerebral and peripheral embolic events. Am J Cardiol 1992; 70:668–72.
7. Daniel WG. Transcatheter closure of patent foramen ovale. Therapeutic overkill or elegant management for selected patients at risk. Circulation 1992; 86:2013–15.
8. Di Tullio M, Sacco RL, Gopal A, Mohr JP, Homma S. Patent foramen ovale as a risk factor for cryptogenic stroke. Ann Intern Med 1992; 117:461–5.
9. Cabanes L, Mas JL, Cohen A et al. Atrial septal aneurysm and patent foramen ovale as risk factors for cryptogenic stroke in patients less than 55 years of age. A study using transesophageal echocardiography. Stroke 1993; 24:1865–73.

10. Jones EF, Calafiore P, Donnan GA, Tonkin AM. Evidence that patent foramen ovale is not a risk factor for cerebral ischemia in the elderly. Am J Cardiol 1994; 596–9.
11. Steiner MM, Di Tullio MR, Rundek T et al. Patent foramen ovale size and embolic brain imaging findings among patients with ischemic stroke. Stroke 1998; 29:944–8.
12. Webster MV, Chancellor AM, Smith HJ et al. Patent foramen ovale in young stroke patients. Lancet 1998; 2:11–12.
13. Windecker S, Meier B. Percutaneous foramen ovale closure: It can be done but should it? Cathet Cardiovasc Intervent 1999; 47:377–80.
14. Overell JR, Bone I, Lees KR. Interatrial septal abnormalities and stroke: a meta-analysis of case-control studies. Neurology 2000; 55:1172–9.
15. Adams HP. Patent foramen ovale: Paradoxical embolism and paradoxica data. Mayo Clin Proc 2004; 79:15–20.
16. Halperin JL, Fuster V. Patent foramen ovale and stroke-another paradoxical twist. Circulation 2002; 105:2580–2.
17. Blackshear JL. Closure of patent foramen ovale in cryptogenic stroke. Ready if not, here come the trials. J Am Coll Cardiol 2004; 44:759–61.
18. Mas JL, Arquizan C, Lamy C et al. Recurrent cerebrovascular events associated with patent foramen ovale, atrial septal aneurysm, or both. New Engl J Med 2001; 345:1740–6.
19. Homma S, Di Tullio MR, Sacco RL, Mihalatos D, Li Mandri G, Mohr JP. Characteristics of patent foramen ovale associated with cryptogenic stroke. A biplane transesophageal echocardiographic study. Stroke 1994; 25:582–6.
20. Mohr JP, Thompson JLP, Lazar RM et al. For the Warfarin-Aspirin Recurrent Stroke Study Group. A comparison of warfarin and aspirin for the prevention of recurrent ischemic stroke. New Engl J Med 2001; 345:1444–51.
21. Mas JL, Zuber M. Recurrent cerebrovascular events in patients with patent foramen ovale, atrial septal aneursym, or both and cryptogenic stroke or transient ischemic attack. French study Group on Patent Foramen Ovale and Atrial Septal Aneurysm. Am Heart J 1995; 130:1083–8.
22. Bogousslavsky J, Garazi S, Jeanrenaud X, Aebischer N, Van Melle G. Stroke recurrence in patients with patent foramen ovale: the Lausanne Study. Lausanne Stroke with Paradoxal Embolism Study Group. Neurology 1996; 46:1301–5.
23. De Castro S, Cartoni D, Fiorelli M et al. Morphological and functional characteristics of patent foramen ovale and their embolic implications. Stroke 2000; 31:2407–13.
24. Homma S, Sacco RL, DiTullio MR, Sciacca RR, Mohr JP. Effect of medical tratment in stroke patients with patent foramen ovale. Patent foramen ovale in cryptogenic stroke study Circulation 2002; 105:2625–31.
25. Windecker S, Wahl A, Nedeltchev K et al. Comparison of medical treatment with percutaneous closure of patent foramen ovale in patients with cryptogenic stroke. J Am Coll Cardiol 2004; 44:750–8.
26. Bridges ND, Hellenbrand W, Latson L, Filiano J, Newburger JW, Lock JE. Transcatheter closure of patent foramen ovale after presumed paradoxical embolism. Circulation 1992; 86:1902–8.
27. Berger F, Uhlemann F, Nürnberg JH, Haas NA, Lange PE. Transkatheterverschluß des persistierenden Foramen ovale als Möglichkeit zur Vermeidung paradoxer Embolien? Dtsch med Wschr 122(1997):1371–6.
28. Rux S, Keppeler P, Dirks J, Sievert H, Schräder R. Interventioneller Verschluß des persistierenden Foramen ovale bei 71 Patienten mit vermuteten paradoxen Embolien: Ein Vergleich zwischen vier verschiedenen Okklusions-Systemen. J Kardiol 1999; 6:17–22.
29. Hung J, Landzberg MJ, Jenkins KJ et al. Closure of patent foramen ovale for paradoxical emboli: intermediate-term risk of recurrent neurological events following transcatheter device placement. J Am Coll Cardiol 2000; 35:1311–16.
30. Windecker S, Wahl A, Chatterjee T et al. Percutaneous closure of patent foramen ovale in patients with paradoxical embolism. Long-term risk of recurrent thrombembolic events. Circulation 2000; 101:893–8.

31. Butera G, Bini MR, Chessa M, Bedogni F, Onofri M, Carminati M. Transcatheter closure of patent foramen ovale in patients with cryptogenic stroke. Ital Heart J 2001; 2:115–18.
32. Sievert H, Horvath K, Zadan E et al. Patent foramen ovale closure in patients with transient ischemia attack/stroke. J Interv Cardiol 2001; 14:261–6.
33. Du ZD, Cao QL, Joseph A et al. Transcatheter closure of patent foramen ovale in patients with paradoxical embolism: Intermediate-term risk of recurrent neurological events. Cathet Cardiovasc Interv 2002; 55:189–94.
34. Braun MU, Fassbender D, Schoen SP et al. Transcatheter closure of patent foramen ovale in patients with cerebral ischemia. J Am Coll Cardiol 2002; 39:2019–25.
35. Beitzke A, Schuchlenz M, Gamillscheg A, Stein HI, Zartner P. Interventioneller Verschluss von Foramen ovale und Vorhofseptumdefekten nach paradox embolischen Ereignissen. Z Kardiol 2002; 91:693–700.
36. Bruch L, Parsi A, Grad MO et al. Transcatheter closure of interatrial communications for secondary prevention of paradoxical embolism-single-center experience. Circulation 2002; 105:2845–8.
37. Martin F, Sanchez PL, Doherty E et al. Percutaneous transcatheter closure of patent foramen ovale in patients with paradoxical embolism. Circulation 2002; 106:1121–6.
38. Schraeder R. Indication and techniques of transcatheter closure of patent foramen ovale. J Interv Cardiol 2003; 16:543–51.
39. Onorato E, Melzi G, Castelli F et al. Patent foramen ovale with paradoxical embolism: mid-term results of transcatheter closure in 256 patients. J Interv Cardiol 2003; 16:46–50.
40. Khositseh A, Cabalka AK, Sweeny JP et al. Transcatheter Amplatzer closure of atrial septal defects and patent foramen ovale in patients with presumed paradoxical embolism. Mayo Clin Proc 2004; 79:35–41.
41. Braun M, Gliech V, Boscheri A et al. Transcatheter closure of patent foramen ovale (PFO) in patients with paradoxical . Eur Heart J 2004; 25:424–30.
42. Schwerzmann M, Windecker S, Wahl A et al. Percutaneous closure of patent foramen ovale: impact of device design on safety and efficacy. Heart 2004; 90:186–90.
43. Jux C, Bertram H. Thrombus formation on intracardiac devices: a complex issue. J Am Coll Cardiol 2004; 44:1712–13.
44. Anzai H, Child J, Natterson B et al. Incidence of thrombus formation on the CardioSEAL and the Amplatzer closure devices. Am J Cardiol 2004; 93:426–31.
45. Krumsdorf U, Ostermayer S, Billinger K et al. Incidence clinical course of thrombus formation on atrial septal defect and patient foramen ovale closure devices in 1000 consecutive patients. J Am Coll Cardiol 2004; 43:302–9.
46. Divekar A, Gaamangwe T, Shaikh N, Raabe M, Ducas J. Cardiac perforation after device closure of atrial septal defects with the Amplatzer septal occluder. J Am Coll Cardiol 2005; 45:1213–18.
47. Wahl A, Krumsdorf U, Meier B et al. Transcatheter treatment of atrial septal aneurysm associated with patent foramen ovale for prevention of recurrent paradoxical embolism in high-risk patients. J Am Coll Cardiol 2005; 45:377–80.

Index

Page numbers in *italics* refer to tables and figures.